FLU HUNTER

World-leading influenza researchers on *Flu Hunter*:

If Tolkien were a virologist, this is the sort of book he would write. An expansive, global story of adventure, discovery and unexpected encounters with microbes and their hosts. The difference is that this story is true! Robert Webster's book is a vivid description of how determination, astute observation and research have given us a profoundly better understanding of influenza, one of the world's most important infectious disease threats. Although it is one man's account, it also shows the importance of international collaboration in research. Highly recommended to anyone with an interest in infectious diseases, public health or the history of science.

MICHAEL BAKER Professor of Public Health,
Department of Public Health, University of Otago, Wellington

In this very valuable book Rob Webster, mentor to influenza researchers all over the world, describes a lifetime of work on influenza viruses. It is essential reading for scientists and public health policy-makers, and a fascinating insight for the general public, by a man who has been at the centre of it all.

MASATO TASHIRO, Former director, WHO Collaborating Centre for
Reference and Research on Influenza, Tokyo

The marvellous real-life story behind some of the great virological discoveries. This autobiographical account of Robert Webster's lifelong quest to understand influenza virus underlines the importance of serendipity in scientific discovery – being in the right place at the right time, with an open and prepared mind. This important witness account will surely form part of the final record of how the mysteries of influenza were unravelled in the 20th and 21st centuries.

MARIA ZAMBON, Deputy Director National Infection Service,
Public Health England

FLU HUNTER

Unlocking the secrets
of a virus

ROBERT G. WEBSTER

OTAGO

Published by Otago University Press
Level 1, 398 Cumberland Street
Dunedin, New Zealand
university.press@otago.ac.nz
www.otago.ac.nz/press

First published 2018
Copyright © Robert G. Webster
The moral rights of the author have been asserted.

ISBN 978-1-98-853131-1

Editors: Sue Hallas and Erika Büky
Indexer: Diane Lowther
Design/layout: Fiona Moffat

Front cover: Artwork by Sharon Webster
Back cover: Author portrait by Jason Bouldin, 2012

Printed in China through Asia Pacific Offset.

CONTENTS

FOREWORD

Influenza is a respiratory disease that impacts on everyone. When a new influenza virus emerges that is able to be transmitted from person to person, it spreads globally, as a pandemic, usually but not always with high mortality, enormous social disruption and substantial economic cost.

A number of influenza pandemics have been documented through the ages, the most serious of course being the Spanish influenza 1918, now a century ago. Unravelling the way these pandemic viruses evolve has challenged the thinking of the most dedicated virologists from around the world since the first influenza virus was isolated in the 1930s.

I became involved in influenza research in the early 1970s, just after the 1968 Hong Kong pandemic. This was a period of transition from the classical era of virology to the molecular era. Professor Robert Webster from Dunedin, New Zealand, had been a flu researcher for a decade or so and I began closely following his research, in which classical epidemiological investigation combined with the newly evolving molecular laboratory technologies to develop the framework we now use for understanding the evolution and control of influenza viruses of human and animal origin.

His lifetime of research has been an incredible journey that started with expeditions to recover viruses from seabirds in Australia in the early 1960s. This led him to the realisation that influenza viruses circulate readily among seabirds without causing disease, and that indeed the natural ecology of most influenza viruses is among wild aquatic birds. Together with another key discovery – that influenza viruses readily evolve or morph through genetic reassortment – led Rob Webster and the other scientists involved to establish a link between the wild aquatic bird virus reservoirs and human influenza pandemics.

It was the *Smithsonian Magazine* that bestowed the moniker 'Flu Hunter' on Rob Webster (www.smithsonianmag.com/science-nature/the-flu-hunter-107190623/), in recognition of the significance of his discoveries. His fascinating journey is documented in this book, with numerous anecdotal stories of his teams' experiences during their field work, which took them all over the world, interacting with governments and other research organisations on every continent. The stories highlight Rob's passion for his work and the obvious enjoyment and satisfaction that he has derived from a career that has spanned over half a century – and is not over yet.

His work has involved collaboration with many world-leading influenza researchers and it is clear that his humble, natural, non-pretentious persona has been a key to these many successful collaborations. Yet he plays down his own contribution at every turn.

The 1918 Spanish influenza pandemic was undoubtedly the most devastating influenza pandemic to date, and Rob Webster has made it his life's work to find out how and why. He has made a remarkable contribution to our understanding of the evolution of influenza viruses and how to control them.

Could it happen again? Webster's warning is clear: '… it is not only possible, it is just a matter of when.'

Flu Hunter chronicles the career of an outstanding global scientific leader. It is a book that will appeal equally to students and scientists familiar with the field, and lay readers. I heartily commend it to all.

LANCE C. JENNINGS
QSO, PhD, FRCPath, FFSc(RCPA),
Clinical Associate Professor, Isirv Chair
April 2018

CHAPTER 1

EMERGENCE OF THE MONSTER: SPANISH INFLUENZA, 1918

The virus that emerged some time in the late Northern Hemisphere summer of 1918 undoubtedly caused the most deadly influenza that humanity has ever encountered. A perfectly healthy young person at the peak of life would develop a headache and muscle soreness, their body temperature would rise as high as 41.1°C (106°F), and some people would become delirious. The person would be so weak that they would fall down; mahogany-coloured spots would appear on the face, which itself would turn blue or blackish from lack of oxygen; and the person would bleed from the ears and nose. The lungs would fill with blood and the sufferer would essentially drown in their own blood. Of the initial survivors, many would be killed by secondary bacterial pneumonia. Both sexes were equally affected, and pregnant women had a 20 per cent probability of miscarriage. In a smaller percentage of survivors, the virus may have spread to the brain, causing delirium and possibly Parkinson's disease or encephalitis lethargica (sleeping sickness) many years later.

Although we do not know where the 'monster strain' of 1918 influenza began, World War I provided the ideal conditions for its development. By September 1918, trenches stretched across Europe from the border of Switzerland to the North Sea. Tens of thousands of soldiers on both sides of the conflict lived half underground, in cramped and often wet conditions. Hygiene was essentially non-existent, with pit latrines and scant washing facilities, and lice and rats as constant irritants (Figure 1.1).

The 1918 influenza came in three waves, the first beginning in March 1918, the second in September to November and the third in early 1919.[1] The first, early in the year, was the mildest. Sufferers experienced the sudden onset of severe headaches, general muscle soreness, and fever with temperatures rising to 38.3–38.9°C (102–103°F). In most infected people, the illness lasted only about four days, but some developed pneumonia, and some died.

While this was a so-called mild wave of the disease, it had an enormous impact on trench warfare. In May 1918 the French army was removing 1500–2000 infected men per day from the front line to the rear. This meant not only that there were fewer soldiers at the front but also that all available transportation was filled, and roads and hospitals were clogged. The situation was similar for the British, Italian and German armies.

This mild strain had in fact been brought to Europe by American troops in early April 1918: unwittingly, the United States had introduced biological warfare into World War I. The German commander Erich von Ludendorff attributed the failure of the German army in the concluding battles of the war not to the superiority of the American troops and their equipment but to the influenza that the American doughboys had brought to the front lines and spread to the German troops. This is quite conceivable: the trenches of the opposing sides were only 30 metres apart in some places, and the virus may have blown across or, more likely, been spread by captured soldiers.

At least a portion of the American troops would have been exposed to this influenza virus earlier and might well have been immune, for it was first described in the small town of Haskell, Kansas, in late February 1918.[2] It was spread by recruits to Camp Funston at Fort

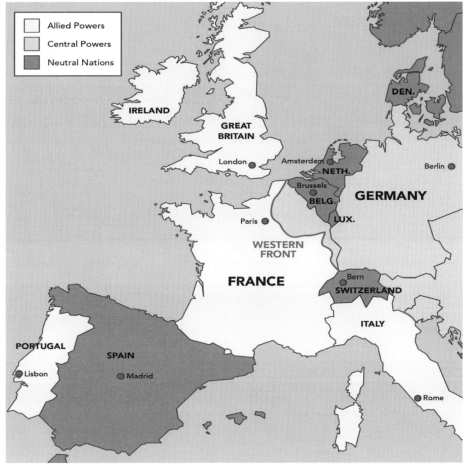

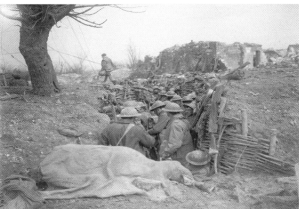

Figure 1.1 Trench warfare in World War I. By 1918 the trenches stretched from the North Sea to the Swiss border. Soldiers fought from trenches dug deeply into the soil, and combatants on both sides were subject to poison-gas clouds.

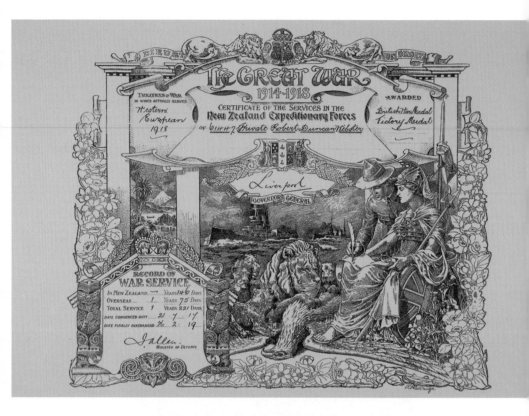

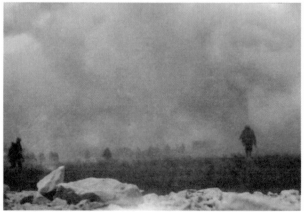

Figure 1.2 Robert Duncan Webster, my father, fought with the New Zealand Expeditionary Forces in the trenches in France, and was wounded in the 100-day offensive in 1918. Like many soldiers, he experienced the deadly gas cloud.

Riley, west of Kansas City, where the camp hospital received its first influenza case on 4 March 1918. Within three weeks, 1100 soldiers were hospitalised. The virus spread rapidly between military camps and to nearby towns, first to Camps Forest and Greenleaf in Georgia, where up to 10 per cent of soldiers were reported sick.[3]

It was inevitable that the ships carrying the first deployment of American troops to Europe would have the virus on board. These vessels were carrying twice as many soldiers as they were designed for, with men sleeping two to a bunk in shifts – ideal conditions for the virus to spread. Because neither the severity nor the fatality rate was particularly high, however, no alarm bells sounded. But in August and September of that year, a second, 'killer' strain of influenza emerged on the return voyages to the United States, turning shipboard life into what was described as 'Hades of Hell', with soldiers vomiting blood.[4] Nevertheless, the American fleet had a lower mortality rate than any other American military group – 6.43 per cent among the troops and 1.5 per cent among the crew – probably because of their earlier exposure to the first wave of influenza.

Besides the horrendous overcrowding and poor hygiene in the trenches of Europe in 1918, there is another reason to believe that the trenches were the probable site of the emergence of the monster strain of 1918 influenza. There was widespread use of poisonous gases, which not only affected the troops directly but could also have caused the influenza virus to mutate and become more lethal.

Despite the Hague Convention of 1907 banning the use of chemical weapons in warfare, poisonous gases were used by both sides in World War I. Since Germany had the largest chemical industry, it is not surprising that it was the heaviest user, but it was not alone. The usage peaked when influenza was circulating among soldiers at the front line. The main chemical agents included chlorine gas, phosgene gas and mustard gas. Although the chemical weapons were not often lethal, they debilitated the troops, causing blisters, blindness and respiratory problems. Incoming supply lines of ammunition, food and fresh troops were blocked by the large numbers of blind and wounded men being led to the rear of the battle zones. Chlorine gas was also an effective psychological weapon – the sight of an incoming cloud of gas became a source of dread to the infantry. My own father was one of the soldiers who experienced the fearful gas cloud (Figure 1.2).

Both phosgene and mustard gas are known mutagenic agents, substances that can cause cells to make mistakes when replicating their DNA. In the laboratory we use mutagenic agents to deliberately change an influenza virus in order to understand the genetic code responsible for reduced or increased disease potential. In the trenches the exposure of virus-infected soldiers to mustard gas could have had the same effect, converting the virus from a relatively mild influenza strain into a killer. Trenches full of thousands of debilitated men would have been the perfect breeding ground for such a virus once it had emerged.[5]

While we will never know exactly where the mutated killer strain of the virus emerged, once it did, it spread quickly to combatants on both sides of the conflict, back down the supply chains to people in nearby towns and cities and then around the world. During the closing battles of World War I, both sides were badly affected. During the milder wave, 10 to 25 per cent of the French troops had to be evacuated from the front line; during the severe wave, the figure rose to 46 per cent. The German war machine was badly affected too.

News of outbreaks of infection among soldiers, sailors and military support personnel was kept quiet by both sides for tactical reasons, with the result that members of the public were deliberately kept in the dark about this imminent threat to their own welfare. It was considered unpatriotic to write anything that might impede the war effort. This code of secrecy extended from public officials to newspapers to the top levels of government and the military. President

Woodrow Wilson, who was kept informed of the outbreaks from March 1918 onwards, was persuaded that news of the death rates on troopships en route to Europe had to be kept quiet so as not to jeopardise the war effort.

The milder influenza hit the headlines in late May 1918, when King Alfonso XIII of Spain and his cabinet members became infected. Since Spain was neutral in World War I, there were no restrictions on publishing this information. The outbreak was reported in Madrid's newspapers as not severe, lasting about four days with no deaths. In October, however, Spain was hit with the second strain and its high mortality rate.[6] Because these first reports of the outbreak occurred in Spain, the pandemic (worldwide epidemic) that ensued was dubbed Spanish influenza.

The Treaty of Versailles, which ended World War I and specified the reparations to be paid to the Allied nations by Germany, was signed in Paris in April 1919. At this conference the 'Big Four' (the prime ministers of France, Britain and Italy and the president of the United States) called the shots. President Wilson wanted Germany to be allowed to retain some resources to aid its economic recovery, but Georges Clemenceau of France ('the Tiger') wanted Germany severely and humiliatingly punished. Wilson threatened to walk out, and then, at the most critical stage of negotiations, he contracted the influenza virus. His young aide, Donald Ferry, was infected on 3 April and died four days later. The president's wife, daughter and other aides were also severely affected. President Wilson survived but with a markedly changed personality. It is possible that the virus damaged his brain; this was one of the sequelae of the monster virus. From his sickbed, Woodrow Wilson capitulated to all of Clemenceau's demands regarding German reparations,[7] which saw Germany sink into a severe economic depression. Whether Wilson's infection was the cause of his changed stance cannot be known.

The worldwide death toll from the Spanish influenza was reported as between 24.7 and 39.3 million but may have been as high as 100 million. The societal disruption and population reduction worldwide were catastrophic.

TWO DISTANT CITIES, TWO APPROACHES

The terrifying impact of the second wave of Spanish influenza was similar in widely disparate places around the world. Events in Philadelphia, Pennsylvania, in the United States, and in Auckland, New Zealand, serve to illustrate the similarities.

Philadelphia

The virus arrived in the port city of Philadelphia on 7 September 1918 with 300 sailors from Boston. The severe strain had surfaced in Boston on 27 August 1918; it was thought to have been brought back from Brest, France. Medical facilities in Philadelphia were quickly overwhelmed, and severely ill sailors began to die: one on the first day, 11 on the second; then the nurse who had tended the first sailor died, and the virus seeded the city.

A huge Liberty Loan parade to raise millions of dollars to support the war effort had been scheduled for 28 September, and despite dire warnings from university and military health officials about the risk of the disease spreading in the crowds, the event went ahead. The parade of sailors, soldiers, marines, boy scouts and women's auxiliary organisations stretched for three kilometres, with thousands watching. Two days later the 31 hospitals in Philadelphia were overflowing with the sick and dying.

By 1 October, three days after the parade, 117 people were dead. All public gatherings were banned, and emergency hospitals were set up. Ten days after the parade, hundreds were dying every day, with thousands afflicted. Symptoms included nosebleeds, cyanosis and delirium. As the supply of coffins ran out, bodies were banked up at funeral homes, and more bodies decayed in houses.

The onslaught peaked in the week of 19 October, when over 4500 people died. Then the death toll declined quite rapidly, and by 25 October the emergency hospitals began to close down. Schools reopened on 28 October. A false report of armistice with Germany on 7 November brought huge crowds hugging and kissing onto the streets of Philadelphia, but there was no resurgence of influenza. The huge celebration was repeated on Armistice Day, 11 November, and once more there was no renewed outbreak.

Researchers in Philadelphia isolated a bacterium, *Haemophilus influenzae*, from the lungs of sufferers and believed this to be the cause of the deadly disease. A vaccine based on the bacterium was developed by health officials and released on 19 October: over 10,000 doses were given to city services personnel. Since the vaccine was given during the waning phase of the pandemic, it appeared effective. It probably also served to calm the fears of the community. But over the 27 weeks of the pandemic, more than 15,700 people died in Philadelphia, with the highest death toll in the 25–34 age group.

Auckland

On the other side of the world in Auckland, New Zealand, the introduction, spread and severity of the highly deadly 1918 Spanish influenza were similar in many ways. The introduction of the virus to New Zealand is controversial. The steamship *Niagara*, which carried New Zealand Prime Minister William Massey home from an imperial war conference in mid-October 1918, has long been blamed for bringing in the virulent strain of influenza. However, influenza cases on board the *Niagara* were immediately quarantined on arrival, so it seems unlikely they could have been responsible for the eventual widespread pandemic. More likely, some now attest, that the hundreds of servicemen returning that month from Europe brought in the monster virus. Most were coming from camps in southern England where the second wave of influenza had been rampant, and on arrival they dispersed throughout the country.[8]

Since no viruses were isolated at that time it is not possible to know for sure; we can only speculate based on written reports. We do know that influenza causing pneumonia and deaths occurred in Auckland and Christchurch on 6 and 8 October, 'with six deaths in the three days before the [*Niagara's*] arrival' on 12 October.[9]

A contributing factor to the spread of the deadly virus in Auckland was that on 8 November a cable arrived indicating that Germany had signed an armistice agreement and the war was over. Aucklanders went berserk with excitement, and the streets were thronged with celebrating citizens. People even left their sickbeds to join in. But the report was incorrect, and city officials closed the pubs and dispersed the crowds. The Spanish influenza pandemic peaked in Auckland four days later, on Armistice Day. There was no public celebration, and 83 people died that day.

City undertakers were overwhelmed. Furniture vans, drapery vans, and horses and carts were commandeered to collect the dead. Victoria Park served as an open-air morgue. As in Philadelphia, healthy young adults were most severely affected, while children seemed to be almost immune. Between 13 and 20 November, two death trains per day moved the dead to the Waikumete Cemetery in West Auckland. By the end of November the death toll in Auckland had fallen to fewer than 10 per day. Church services resumed after 4 December, and city services returned to normal.

Overall, 1021 people died in Auckland – a death rate of 7.6 per thousand. City health officials used zinc sulphate aerosol spray as a preventative, although bringing people together for treatment probably contributed to the disease's spread rather than its prevention.

These two cities were by no means the worst affected by the 1918 Spanish influenza, which invaded almost the entire world (though strict quarantine efforts managed to keep the virulent strain out of American Samoa). Some communities were more severely affected than others: among the native peoples of Alaska, almost the entire adult population died.

A hundred years on from one of the greatest disease pandemics in recorded history, we can ask, what did the 1918 Spanish influenza teach us? There are many lessons:

- Influenza is variable in severity, and we still cannot accurately predict whether an outbreak will be severe.

- Although more young adults died in 1918 than young children and older people, the opposite was the case in the influenza pandemics of 1957 (H2N2) and 1968 (H3N2), but the milder 2009 (H1N1) pandemic again showed an age-based mortality similar to the 1918 (H1N1) pandemic, showing that different strains affect age groups differently.

- Influenza spreads more rapidly in crowded conditions.

- Some segments of the world's population are more susceptible than others.

- Infection with a mild influenza virus can provide protection from a severe wave of the same strain.

- Quarantine can be effective but is extremely difficult to implement.

- Bacterial infection following influenza can be a major contributor to high mortality.

- Face masks can provide some protection and delay infection.

- Zinc sulphate aerosols do not provide protection.

- An analgesic (aspirin) effectively treats fever.

What health officials did not know in 1918 was the cause of influenza. Nor did they know how a mild strain of influenza could become a killer, or what medicines and vaccines could help. The rest of this book offers my personal insights into these questions from a lifetime of research. It illustrates how advances in science are part hard work and part good luck, along with a willingness to accept rejection and failure, and to get your hands dirty. It has been the most rewarding career imaginable.

CHAPTER 2

THE START OF
INFLUENZA RESEARCH

After the deadly outbreak of Spanish influenza, health authorities dreaded what would happen next. Would this monster virus continue to circulate, or would it revert to a milder form of influenza? Public health officials worldwide began to investigate these questions through research that one day would lead to the development of suitable vaccines.

The years that followed the 1918 outbreak saw sporadic, severe outbreaks in different parts of the world. In 1920 there were 11,000 influenza deaths in Chicago and New York City, with the latter reporting more influenza deaths in one day that year than on any single day in 1918. On the other side of the world, Australia had enforced the quarantining of ships and had succeeded in keeping out the severe wave until 1919, when it struck and caused societal disruption. However, overall, there were fewer deaths that year (2.3 deaths per 1000 people) than in New Zealand in 1918 (5.8/1000).[10] Severe sporadic outbreaks continued through 1919, 1920 and 1921, but by 1922 influenza had declined in severity and returned to so-called ordinary or seasonal influenza.

Ordinary influenza today is similar to – if probably slightly milder than – the influenza of the first wave in 1918. It begins suddenly with headaches, chills, a non-productive cough, fever with temperatures of 38–40°C (100.4–106°F), muscle aches, general weakness and loss of appetite. The fever is usually gone after three days, but general weakness can last up to two weeks. There is a tendency to trivialise seasonal influenza, but in New Zealand it kills 400 people a year in a population of 4.7 million.[11]

The average direct medical costs of an annual epidemic and the wider economic burden in New Zealand are currently being measured but are estimated to run into the billions of dollars. In the US, on average, 35,000 people die per year in a population of 320 million (based on a 2007 analysis).[12] The average direct medical cost for an annual epidemic is US$10.4 billion and the economic burden $87.1 billion. Thus seasonal influenza is not a trivial disease by any measure. People are well advised to be vaccinated annually with the vaccine formulation recommended by the World Health Organization (WHO). National recommendations vary regarding which age groups should be vaccinated.

In the decades after the 1918 Spanish influenza pandemic, the virus responsible – the H1N1 influenza virus – continued to evolve. It caused annual epidemics in humans in the winter months in temperate latitudes and year-round epidemics in the tropics. In 1957 another major change occurred. A different strain of the influenza virus (H2N2) emerged in Asia, causing the second pandemic of the twentieth century, which killed 1.5 million people. In 1968 came the H3N2 virus, which caused the Hong Kong pandemic. The return of the H1N1 virus caused pandemics in 1977 and 2009. A timeline of the epidemics and pandemics of influenza in the past century is shown in Figure 2.1.

There are three types of influenza virus, labelled A, B and C. A fourth type, D, has also been proposed. Type A is found in humans, lower animals and birds; type B is found mainly in humans but has been detected in seals too; type C is found mainly in human children and pigs; and type D is found in bovines. Type A influenza viruses are the ones that cause epidemics and pandemics in humans, including the Spanish influenza of 1918. There are 16 subtypes of influenza A found in aquatic birds and two subtypes recently discovered in bats.

One of the main features of influenza viruses, amply demonstrated during the 1918 pandemic, is that they are extremely variable. The 1918 virus changed from a mild to a deadly virus and then back to mild. What is the secret of this variability? Why does the virus succeed in causing epidemics and pandemics again and again?

As with all disease agents, there is a constant battle between the attacking virus and the host. As the influenza virus attaches to the cell lining of the nose, throat and lungs, the body responds by releasing an array of protective chemicals (cytokines), followed by antibodies that attach specifically to the invading virus so that scavenging macrophages (white blood cells with a 'clean-up' function) can remove it. (The virus molecules to which the antibodies attach are known as antigens.) In addition, the body makes killer cells designed to destroy the virus. During this clash, the body temperature rises, and the person begins experiencing the characteristic aches and pains of influenza, due in part to the rather toxic chemicals produced by the human body to kill the virus. Within a week, the body has usually won the battle, the person recovers, and the body keeps a immunological memory of the invader in its protective arsenal, ready to deploy more antibodies if the virus attacks again.

Despite the body's ability to augment its protective arsenal in this way, the virus is sometimes able to overcome these defences because it can change its surface configuration so that the body no longer recognises it as familiar. There are two ways in which the virus can change. During their multiplication, influenza viruses continually make errors in assembling their genetic building blocks. There is no quality control in the process, so a mixture of viruses is

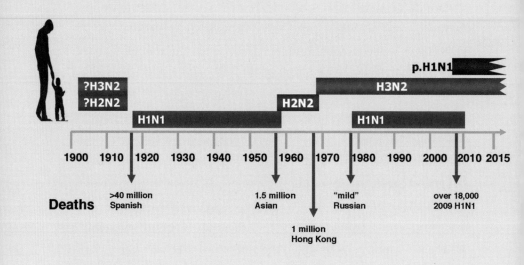

Figure 2.1 Influenza epidemics and pandemics of the past century. (A pandemic is an epidemic that spreads to humans all over the world.) Pandemics occurred in 1918 (HINI Spanish), in 1957 (H2N2 Asian), in 1968 (H3N2 Hong Kong), in 1977 (HINI Russian) and in 2009 (HINI). After the emergence of each new pandemic strain, that virus causes epidemics until a new pandemic emerges.

Figure 2.2 (opposite) The surface of an influenza particle is covered in three kinds of projections. The most frequent is the club-shaped haemagglutinin (H) spike (shown in purple), which attaches the virus to docking sites on cells of the human nose, throat and lungs. The second is the neuraminidase (N) spike (pink), an enzyme that serves as molecular scissors to free the virus from the cell surface and facilitate virus spread. The third spike (M2) is a tube-like structure (yellow). Each of these projections is embedded in a lipid (fatty) layer that the virus steals from the human cell as it buds off from that cell. Inside the lipid layer, a membrane (M) protein (white) surrounds the eight RNA segments that contain the virus genetic information.

produced, some like the parent virus and many with genetic changes that make it different from the parent. When this mixture of viruses infects a person with antibody memory, the variant influenza viruses circumvent the host's immune response because they have antigens that the immune system does not recognise. This change in genetic material is called 'drift' or 'genetic drift', and it is how seasonal or ordinary influenza changes from year to year. As the human population becomes resistant to the prevailing virus, variants with errors survive and cause the next epidemic.

The second phenomenon that yields viral variety is known as 'reassortment' (hybridisation), a process by which two influenza viruses mix their gene segments, a bit like mating. An influenza virus has eight separate RNA segments of genetic information (Figure 2.2). When two different influenza A viruses infect the same cell, it is possible to generate 256 genetically distinct offspring. This is the process that led to the emergence of most of the human influenza pandemics in the twentieth century.

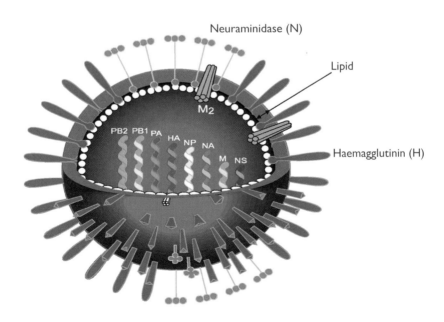

WHAT IS A VIRUS?

A virus is the ultimate parasite – an obligate intracellular parasite, meaning that it is totally dependent on the living cells of hosts for its existence. It is a tiny piece of genetic information (RNA or DNA) wrapped in a protein overcoat. Viruses infect every class of living organism, including plants, animals and bacteria, often but not always causing disease. There are more viruses in the world than any other biological entity. In the computer age, the term is used to describe commands that replicate themselves and spread extensively, causing disruption (disease), as occurs with biological viruses.

Viruses are the smallest organisms known.

Influenza is caused by an RNA virus that has eight separate pieces of genetic information that permit it to hybridise with influenza viruses of the same type.

Influenza viruses are about 100 nanometres (nm) in diameter (a human hair is 80,000–100,000nm) and vary in shape from spherical to filamentous. The component parts of the virus are made by the infected human cell's machinery under instructions from the virus's genetic code. The components are then inserted into the lipid (fatty) membrane that surrounds the cell, turning that membrane into the outer shell of the virus. The end result is a virus particle with a shell sporting a layer of club-like projections or spikes. There are three kinds of spike, the most numerous of which is haemagglutinin (H). This attaches the virus to receptors (docking sites) on human cells. The second type of spike, neuraminidase (N), occurs in clumps. This enzyme acts like molecular scissors and clips the surface of a cell to free the virus, enabling it to spread. The third spike is the matrix 2 protein, a short, tube-like projection. Under the lipid layer, there is a matrix (M) layer that surrounds the eight RNA segments that make up the viral genetic code.

The naming of influenza viruses was standardised by the WHO in 1980. Each name includes the type of virus, the animal host from which the virus was isolated (by convention, humans are not specified), the country, the isolate number and the year. In parentheses are the haemagglutinin and neuraminidase subtypes. For example, A/Madrid/101/1918 (H1N1) would be an influenza A virus isolated from a human in Madrid, isolate number 101 from 1918, the H subtype and N subtype being H1N1. If the influenza virus had been isolated from a pig, the name would be A/swine/Madrid/101/1918 (H1N1).

In 1919–20, public health officials in New Zealand, Britain, the US and other countries undertook major reviews of the medical understanding of influenza. There was general agreement that if a vaccine was to be developed, research on the nature of the causative agent was urgently needed.

When *Haemophilus influenzae* bacteria were isolated from the throats of infected people during the 1918 pandemic, the consensus among scientists was that these bacteria were the cause of the disease, hence the name. This conclusion was supported by studies showing that vaccines prepared from these bacteria appeared to be effective. The timing of vaccine administration (during the pandemic's waning phase) was bound to lend support to this notion. In fact, the vaccines probably did provide some protection against the bacterium and the secondary pneumonia it caused – a major cause of death during the pandemic. The bacteria were not, however, the primary cause of influenza.

The first clue that the causative agent was a virus came from an unexpected and completely unappreciated source. In 1901 two Italian scientists, Eugenio Centanni and Ezio Savonuzzi, showed that the highly lethal disease of chickens known as fowl plague was caused by a nonbacterial agent, one of the first pathogens to be classified as a virus.[13] Fowl plague is a disease that begins in the nasal tract and lungs of chickens and spreads through the blood to every tissue in the body, including the brain. Up to 100 per cent of infected birds die, with haemorrhages in all organs. But the characteristics of fowl plague were so different from those of human influenza that no connection was suspected. It was not until 1955 that Werner Schäfer from Tubingen, Germany, showed a relationship between the fowl plague and human viruses.[14]

Meanwhile, John S. Koen, a veterinarian in the US Department of Agriculture at Fort Dodge, Iowa, reported in 1918 that a respiratory disease breaking out in pigs was remarkably similar to the influenza appearing in humans.[15] In 1928, transmission studies with unfiltered mucus from infected pigs enabled Charles S. McBryde at the Bureau of Animal Industry to transmit influenza from pig to pig. However, he failed to transmit the disease using mucus passed through a bacteria-proof filter, which was a criterion for identifying a virus at the time. Because viruses are smaller than bacteria, this type of filtration provided the earliest way to distinguish between bacteria and viruses. A few years later Richard E. Shope of the Rockefeller Institute for Medical Research in New York repeated the filtration studies and successfully transmitted influenza between pigs, formally showing that the causative agent was a virus.[16]

At this time the Medical Research Council (MRC) of Britain was also conducting research on viruses. Since distemper in dogs was affecting the English sport of foxhunting, the magazine *The Field* gave the MRC generous funding to study the problem. Distemper in dogs begins with a high fever and cough, vomiting and diarrhoea. The dogs develop fits of paralysis and often die. Patrick Laidlaw, who headed the laboratory, had heard that ferrets caught distemper from dogs and in 1921 set up a strict isolation laboratory at Mill Hill Laboratories outside London to study the disease.[17]

Christopher Andrewes, a young biologist from the MRC, had just spent two years studying rheumatic fever at the Rockefeller Institute, where Shope had studied swine influenza, and had established a friendship with Shope. After Andrewes returned to the MRC, this rather loose professional network came to the fore during a sudden outbreak of seasonal influenza in London in 1933. Andrewes, Laidlaw and their colleague Wilson Smith collected throat samples from influenza patients and, using Shope's methods, successfully infected ferrets (a good model for investigating influenza because they show the same symptoms of infection as humans). They also showed that the agent was filterable and therefore met the definition of a virus. They also fulfilled Koch's postulates for identifying the causative agent of a disease, which require isolation of the agent in pure culture, evidence that the isolated agent causes disease when introduced into a healthy animal, and re-isolation of the same agent from the infected animal. Their work proved that a viral agent did cause the disease.

During the ferret transmission studies, a ferret had sneezed on Charles Stuart-Harris, a medical student in Smith's laboratory, who went on to develop influenza symptoms. The agent was isolated from Stuart-Harris and transmitted back to ferrets, then re-isolated from the animals.[18] Back at the Rockefeller Institute, Shope had repeated the ferret studies and noted that it was much easier to infect ferrets if they had first been anaesthetised allowing the virus to be inserted deep into the lungs to contact susceptible cells. This information provided the breakthrough to the team in London, who had moved on from ferrets and had been trying (without success) to infect laboratory mice. Thomas Francis at the Rockefeller Institute also succeeded in infecting mice with influenza under anaesthesia, and thereafter the mouse became the standard laboratory animal for influenza studies, because they are small and easy to breed.

The next big challenge for influenza research was finding a simple way to isolate and grow the viruses. Researchers at the MRC laboratories in London were having limited success in growing the virus in chicken eggs. The method involved getting a 10-day-old developing egg, drilling a hole in the shell and injecting it with a throat wash from an influenza-infected person. Frank MacFarlane Burnet from Australia contributed to this work during his two-year fellowship at the MRC. After his return to Melbourne he discovered that if the samples from the human influenza patients were injected into the liquid-filled amniotic cavity that surrounds the chicken embryo, the influenza virus multiplied quite well.[19] The MRC team also found that on subsequent passaging (injecting the fluid from the first egg into a second egg, then into a third egg), the virus would multiply well when injected into the much larger allantoic cavity of the 10–12-day-old chicken embryo.

This readily available source of virus quickly led to the discovery that allantoic fluid containing the virus would agglutinate red blood cells from chickens or humans (cause them to stick together).[20] The property of haemagglutination by influenza viruses could be quantified and so provided a simple method for measuring the amount of virus present. Importantly, the reaction was inhibited by serum from people who had recovered from an influenza infection. So, a simple serological assay, the haemagglutination inhibition test, allowed researchers to compare different isolates of influenza virus and determine a vaccine's efficacy. George Hirst also noticed that haemagglutination of red blood cells by influenza viruses was not permanent and proposed that the virus possessed an enzyme that released it from the red blood cells.[21] This astute observation led to the eventual identification of the neuraminidase enzyme on the surface of influenza viruses and to a second serological test for influenza.[22]

These developments soon led to the isolation of a completely different type of influenza virus, designated type B.[23] This new strain was isolated at the Rockefeller Institute by Thomas Francis and sent to the team in London for verification. These two groups could show no relationships between the antigens of earlier strains and those of the new isolate, and they agreed to call the original 'type A influenza virus' and the new strain 'type B influenza virus'.

Willingness to share information and virus strains has always been a feature of influenza research. The first network of influenza scientists in New York, London and Melbourne developed much of the early knowledge about the virus by sharing freely. With the inception of the WHO in 1947, influenza was recognised as a continuing global health problem, one that was complicated by the antigenic variations of the virus from year to year. Andrewes (later Sir Christopher) proposed to the WHO the need for a global network for influenza research and the designation of reference laboratories. Scientists in the existing informal international network agreed, and the WHO collaborating network was established in 1952, when 26 laboratories contributed their influenza isolates.

Andrewes' own laboratories at Mill Hill were designated the World Influenza Centre. Other collaborating centres were established in Melbourne, Atlanta, Tokyo, Memphis and later in Beijing. National laboratories in any country that wished to participate in the network could send their influenza virus isolates to the designated collaborating laboratory in their region, which would characterise the influenza and send them the results. The collaborating laboratories (known as reference laboratories) prepared sera in ferrets to identify the circulating influenza viruses and provided standardised methods for isolating and identifying them. This information was shared between the centres, facilitating the updating of vaccines.[24] Since 1973 the key staff from all collaborating centre laboratories have met to decide on the changes to make to human vaccines to cope with antigenic drift, and WHO has provided a formal recommendation on the strains to include in the vaccine.

The Global Influenza Surveillance Network (GISN) was founded in 1952 and expanded to the Global Influenza Surveillance and Response System (GISRS) in 2011. It currently consists of 152 institutions, including 143 national influenza centres in 113 countries. The influenza WHO network was the prototype for all the other networks that have been subsequently developed by the WHO.

The influenza network faced its first real challenge in 1957, when the second influenza pandemic of the twentieth century emerged in Yunnan Province in southern China. The causative virus was completely different from previous strains yet was still an influenza A virus.[25] Fortunately, by 1957 it was known that the causative agent was a virus and that vaccines could be prepared in chicken eggs. The question at that time was whether human influenza pandemics emerged as a result of the great variability of the circulating human influenza virus or whether they were coming from animal sources such as pigs or chickens.

CHAPTER 3

FROM SEABIRDS IN AUSTRALIA TO TAMIFLU

Scientific knowledge can be advanced in many ways, and a major development in the search for the origin of pandemic influenza viruses came from a walk on the beach I took in 1967 with the late Graeme Laver. In 2004 he wrote:

> The story started in the late 1960s on the south coast of New South Wales in Australia. We noticed that every 10 to 15 m or so there were some dead muttonbirds (shearwaters) washed up on the beach. Knowing that terns in South Africa had been killed by an influenza virus in 1961,[26] we wondered if these birds too had died from a flu infection.[27]

The name 'muttonbirds' here refers to the migratory seabirds *Puffinus pacificus*, which fly on a figure-8 route around the Pacific Ocean and return yearly to nest and raise their young on small islands south of New Zealand and on the Great Barrier Reef islands of Australia. Their common name derives from the fact that in New Zealand these birds served as a ready source of meat for Māori and early European settlers because plump, juicy young birds could be easily pulled from their shallow burrows. Muttonbirds have a dense layer of rich, fishy-tasting fat just under the skin, and they have traditionally been salted and smoked. In recent years they have become a New Zealand delicacy at gourmet restaurants. Laver and I decided that it would be a bit of lark to head to the muttonbird nesting sites on the Great Barrier Reef, on a hunch that they might indeed be infected with influenza.

At that time, I was a graduate student at the Australian National University (ANU) in Canberra, and Laver was a newly recruited junior scientist there. We had no resources to finance this proposed expedition. The islands on the Great Barrier Reef are protected, so we needed to obtain permission for an expedition, and we would also have to lug in all the water, food and equipment we needed by boat. We approached the head of the Department of Microbiology in ANU's John Curtin School for Medical Research, whose response was 'You have to be joking! Scientific expedition, my foot. More like a junket to take your friends and families on another of your outback adventures.'

He was largely right, but we did not give up. We knew that Martin Kaplan, head of the Veterinary Virology section of the WHO, was a strong proponent of the theory that swine were a possible source of pandemic influenza in humans, so we took our idea to him. To our delight, Kaplan approved US$500 for the expedition. Back in the late 1960s, $500 was a substantial award that would indeed cover most of the costs. The ANU then reconsidered and decided that there was a scientific aspect to the expedition after all. They agreed to provide one vehicle (a station wagon) and fuel for transportation to and from our chosen port. Participants from ANU came in their own vehicles. The port offering the easiest access to the uninhabited islands where the muttonbirds bred was Gladstone, north of Brisbane in Queensland, some 1500 kilometres by road from Canberra.

Our final destinations were Tryon, North West and Lady Elliot Islands. These are sandy cays with scrubby vegetation but no fresh water. In the days before easy radio or any kind of digital

---

Figure 3.1 (opposite) Our search for influenza viruses in birds took us to the islands of the Great Barrier Reef in Australia. This map shows our route from Canberra to Gladstone, the nearest port giving access to reef. Inset photos show (top to bottom):

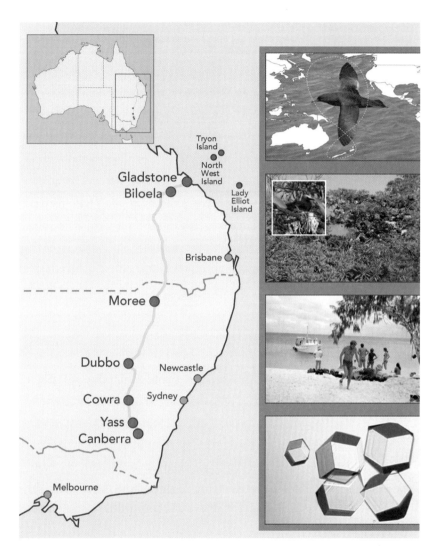

a) The 'figure 8' migration route of shearwaters (muttonbirds, *Puffinus pacificus*) around the Pacific Ocean. The birds breed and raise their young in shallow burrows on the islands south of New Zealand and the islands of the Great Barrier Reef of Australia.

b) Noddy terns are resident on North West Island. We caught adult birds for sampling directly from their nests; having never seen humans they were unafraid of us.

c) Dr Graeme Laver (in red trunks) and the research party arriving on Tryon Island.

d) Crystals of the neuraminidase (N) prepared by Graeme Laver from the H1N9 influenza virus isolated from a noddy tern and used in the design of the anti-influenza drug Tamiflu.

communication, we had to be prepared to be completely self-sufficient for up to two weeks on the islands. That meant bringing 7.5 litres of fresh water per person per day, along with a lot of food, and bird sampling supplies, including Dacron swabs and a large insulated thermos flask (known as a Dewar flask) of liquid nitrogen for keeping samples cold.

There was no shortage of volunteers for the expedition: colleagues from Germany, England and the US raised their hands. We usually had 10–12 participants. Preference was given to families with teenage children, who had the advantage of being lighter than adults and so would be less likely to break through the shallow sand burrows of the muttonbirds and squash them (Figure 3.1).

The organisation of the first expedition served as the model for the subsequent seven field trips that followed at one- or two-year intervals. After assembling all of the scientific supplies and loading them into the vehicles, the team set out in convoy for the two-day trip from Canberra to Gladstone. We followed the inland rather than coastal route to bypass the major cities of Sydney, Newcastle and Brisbane. Another advantage of the outback road was that we could stop for the night wherever we chose and set up camp right by the road. On one trip there was a plague of mice in that part of Australia, and we had their unwelcome company in our tents at night. It was not much of a problem in a tent with a floor, but very early one morning our German colleagues erupted from their floorless tent, flinging mice out of their sleeping bags and clothing. That mouse plague was quite amazing – at night the surface of the road seemed to shimmer as the rodents moved over it.

The boat trip from Gladstone to Tryon Island was always a challenge: the sea could vary from glassy smooth to wild and barely crossable. I was seriously concerned on one expedition when the captain elected to stay behind and let the first mate take the helm.

It was so rough that even scopolamine patches failed to suppress the motion sickness. Water washed over the boat with its tied-down hatches. Once we entered the coral reefs surrounding the coral cay, however, the sea was calm and the pristine beaches inviting, and our unpleasant sea crossing was soon forgotten. On the initial trip, the supplies were ferried ashore by rowboat, and the launch returned to Gladstone; on later trips the launch stayed with us in the coral lagoon, enabling us to sample birds on many islands in the area.

A large tent for cooking and eating was the centre of activities, and this base tent was set up in the shade of the abundant trees (*Pizonia grandis*). Individual pup tents were pitched nearby for sleeping and housing personal gear. We generally spent the days swimming and snorkelling on the most fabulous coral reef in the world, harvesting fish and lobster for our meals. The evenings were spent doing the science. This schedule, I hasten to point out, was dictated by the birds' behaviour, not just our preferences, since dusk was when the parent birds returned to their burrows with bellies full of fish for their large and rapidly growing juveniles. The rookeries at dusk were a cacophony, with incoming parent birds calling to their impatiently waiting offspring.

After dusk we lit lanterns and walked very carefully into the rookeries. It was the children who usually caught the birds. They would lie on the ground at a burrow that was emitting plenty of 'bird talk' and reach in and pull out the bird, holding its feet and wings. When a new recruit had an arm deep in the burrow, Graeme Laver would invariably say, 'Be careful of the snakes!' In fact there are no snakes in the coral cays, but the warning always brought the same panicked reaction – a rapid withdrawal with no bird. This initiation rite brought laughter each time.

In the early years we took a throat swab and a blood sample (from the wing vein) from each bird and quickly returned it to its burrow.

Later, once we knew that influenza in birds is found in the intestine, we also took a swab from the bird's cloaca (birds have a cloaca, not an anus). The blood was allowed to clot and separate in the sample tubes overnight, and the clear serum was removed and stored in the aforementioned thermos flask, where it was kept frozen (along with the individual swabs). After sampling some 50 to 60 birds, the group would return to the base tent, the adults enjoyed a glass of sherry and we all partook of a sumptuous seafood meal prepared by the designated cook for that day.

Although our colleagues around the world heard only that we were having great fun, day after day of snorkelling and fishing in paradise can actually become boring. Since noddy terns (*Anous tenuirostris*) were also on the islands, we decided to satisfy our vast scientific curiosity by spending the daylight hours sampling them as well.

The expeditions were not without incident, despite some house rules. One rule stipulated the wearing of a hat, shirt and sneakers at all times during daylight hours, including while swimming. The sunshine was intense, and severe sunburn would have been debilitating. Shoes were required because stonefish with toxic spines and razor clams lurked in the sandy shallows. My two children, Nick and Sally, aged 11 and 13 years respectively, joined the third expedition and were unimpressed, deciding early on that I was being an overprotective parent. This changed on the first evening on Tryon Island. A visiting scientist from the Netherlands had ignored the footwear rule and had been enjoying walking along the beautiful coral beach and clear water in bare feet until he stepped on a sharp object and cut his foot deeply. The visitor was very lucky it was not a stonefish. There was no further static about wearing shoes or the other house rules.

That same night we were woken by severe ground tremors and were all very alarmed. The cause turned out to be a giant sea turtle that was under a corner of our tent digging a hole to lay her eggs! We had pitched our tent on her nesting spot, but she claimed it regardless. Once again we were grateful for our tent floor. The digging went on for nearly an hour before the turtle settled down to lay what appeared to be hundreds of eggs, each about the size of a golf ball, with a flexible, leathery skin. Early the next morning Nick got his own back and rode the massive creature for part of her trip back to the ocean. Although the turtle lumbered along the beach, back in the water she was fast and elegant.

Another rule for uninhabited islands is 'Don't swim on an incoming tide' because this is when sharks may enter the lagoon to feed. Our group did get caught out once when we had to wade in chest-deep water back to the launch at North West Island. We had gone there at low tide to catch noddy terns, a relatively easy task since the terns would stay on the nests, unafraid of predators. Our mother ship was some 275 metres off the beach when the captain blew the recall alarm because a storm had suddenly blown in. The children were put into the rowboat while the adults waded, sharks notwithstanding, to the launch on the incoming tide. The sharks must not have been ready to feed, as we made it all in one piece to the launch. I have never been so happy to be on a storm-tossed boat as when we left that island.

On the first Barrier Reef trip, Laver tested the sera of the muttonbirds right on the island. He put the serum into a small hole in a clear gel beside a hole containing killed influenza virus disrupted with detergent. The next day there was a white line between the virus and the muttonbird sera where a component of the virus combined with antibody in the serum to form a precipitate. This meant the serum from the muttonbird contained antibodies to influenza, which meant in turn that at some time in the past the bird had been infected with an influenza virus (the test did not indicate which). Back in the laboratory at ANU, there was more testing to be done.

Being a biochemist, Laver opted to test the muttonbird sera for their ability to block the activity of the neuraminidase enzyme found on the surface of an influenza virus (see Chapter 2). When this enzyme is active, it releases a chemical that turns the indicator bright red; when the activity is blocked (by an antibody), the indicator remains clear. The question was, which virus should he use in the test? Laver chose the virus responsible for the 1957 Asian pandemic, H2N2. In the first batch of muttonbird sera, one of the 20 samples being tested remained clear. Laver described the excitement: 'It was one of those rare "eureka" moments that makes scientific research exhilarating.' The serum from one muttonbird had inhibited the enzyme activity of the human virus, meaning that the bird had previously been infected by an influenza virus related to the human H2N2 influenza virus.

The next step was to isolate the virus itself from the muttonbirds. The initial studies were disappointing: no influenza viruses were isolated from the hundreds of throat swabs taken from the birds. This justified going back to the Barrier Reef and trying again. From the second trip, in 1972, one influenza virus was isolated from the throat swabs of over 200 birds sampled.[28] This virus was different from any virus previously reported in that it possessed a novel form of neuraminidase. It was designated A/Shearwater/Australia/1/72 (H6N5). The virus had come from the throat of an apparently healthy bird and did not cause disease when subsequently inoculated into healthy ducks, chickens and turkeys, even though it multiplied to high levels in the birds.

In the interim, I had moved to St Jude Children's Research Hospital in Memphis, Tennessee. One of the things I was keen to do was examine populations of migratory waterfowl on other continents, such as migratory ducks in Canada.

We know now that the influenza virus in aquatic birds multiplies mainly in the intestinal tract and was spread to other birds by means of faeces excreted into the water.[29] We realised that for years we had been looking at the wrong end of the bird for influenza viruses – the throat instead of the cloaca. From samples collected in 1975 we had isolated eight influenza viruses from apparently healthy noddy terns and one from the throat of a healthy shearwater. Full characterisation of the viruses revealed that the one from the shearwater was related to the H5N3 influenza virus that had killed many terns on the coast of South Africa in 1961. However, the shearwater virus caused no apparent disease, either in the host bird or in our experiments with ducks, chickens and turkeys.

This led to the key finding that harmless versions of influenza viruses can be carried by apparently healthy migratory birds but that the same viruses can undergo changes and become killers. Perhaps the most important of all the viruses isolated from birds on the Barrier Reef was from the 70th cloacal swab of a noddy tern caught on North West Island by Adrian Gibbs. This influenza virus was characterised as an H11N9 and contained a neuraminidase that had not been previously described.

The ultimate goal of our studies was to provide treatments and cures for influenza, but first we had to better understand the origin of the viruses. If we could determine the structure of an influenza virus and its components, a drug to prevent or cure the disease could be developed. So the goal was to find the 'active site' on the neuraminidase molecule, the part that enables it to separate from a host cell and spread through the body. Laver set out to do this by bombarding the molecule with x-rays at a cyclotron in Switzerland.

Although breakthroughs in medicine are often illustrated by images of scientists hunched over microscopes to discover disease agents, molecules are too small to be observed by ordinary visual magnification. One technique for examining them is to place them in a beam of x-rays, which have a much shorter wavelength than visible light. The molecular structure can be determined from the way the molecule diffracts the x-ray beam. However, to use this technique, samples must be prepared in the form of crystals through which the x-ray beam can pass. This typically involves placing the biological sample in a chemical solution (such as a salt solution) under conditions that encourage the formation or 'growth' of crystals, like creating rock candy from a sugar solution.

Growing good crystals is a challenging and delicate task. At the time, Laver was probably the greatest crystal grower in the world. He isolated the N9 neuraminidase from a virus isolated from the noddy tern and set out to grow the best crystals the world had ever seen. One of the techniques at that time, believe it or not, was to send the material into space on a NASA space shuttle, where microgravity allowed large crystals to form. Unfortunately, the *Challenger* explosion in January 1986 brought that method to a halt. Not to be stopped, Laver approached scientists of the Soviet Union and persuaded them to send the influenza neuraminidase protein to the MIR space station. The possibility that the Soviets might achieve a major breakthrough in crystal making worried American strategists, but the plan went ahead. (Laver loved to stir the pot and revelled in creating problems for American and Soviet strategists.)

The strategists need not have worried, however, for the crystals were, at best, only marginally better than those grown on Earth. Some scientists speculated that the re-entry and bump-down of the supply spacecraft in Kazakhstan may not have been beneficial to the crystals, and that perhaps top-quality crystals had indeed been grown on the MIR and then wrecked. Regardless, subsequent advances in robotics enabled the creation of optimal conditions for crystallisation, making it possible to grow large, high-quality crystals safely on Earth.

At the time, an anti-influenza drug called Relenza had been developed based on the structure of the human H2N2 neuraminidase, but it had to be puffed into the respiratory tract of patients, which is not easy. An easier delivery system was needed. Laver provided crystals of the isolated N9 neuraminidase from the noddy tern, H11N9, to Gilead Sciences of California to assist in the design of a drug that could be taken as a pill. The drug now known as Tamiflu was developed by Gilead scientists and was later acquired by the Roche company. It is currently the most widely used drug for treatment of influenza. As Laver pointed out, Tamiflu could have been developed using N2 neuraminidase crystals, but when Gibbs caught the noddy tern whose sample provided the large and near-perfect N9 crystals, it made the job a whole lot easier. So a walk on the beach provided a vital insight into the origin of pandemic influenza viruses and contributed to the development of an important new drug.

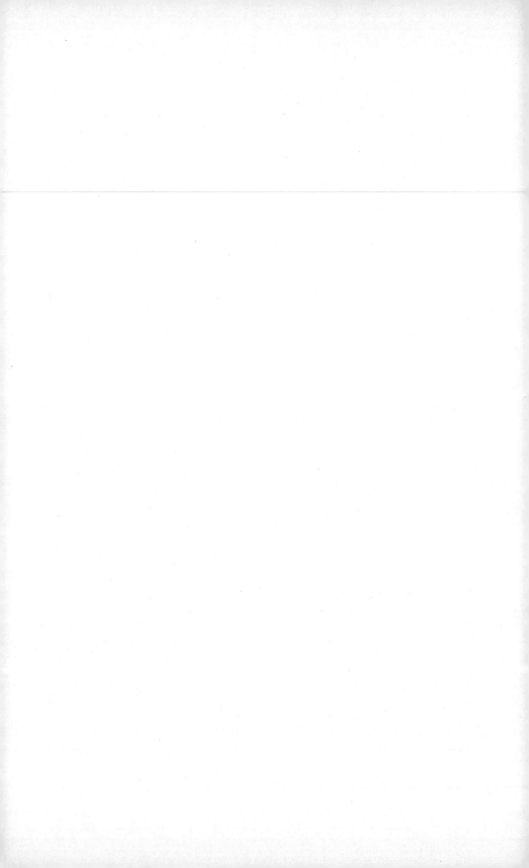

CHAPTER 4

THE SEARCH MOVES TO WILD DUCKS IN CANADA

After our success in isolating influenza viruses from seabirds on the Great Barrier Reef, Graeme Laver and I decided to test whether influenza viruses related to those in humans could be found in other species of birds in other parts of the world. One of the world's largest populations of pelagic (open ocean) birds is found off the coast of Peru and Chile, on the Guano Islands, which had built up from the droppings of millions of seabirds over time and were mined for agricultural fertiliser. Smaller populations of many other gull species and noddy terns also inhabit the Dry Tortugas, islands off the western end of the Florida Keys in the United States. It was these latter populations that we targeted in 1974, using the techniques honed on the Great Barrier Reef. Over a thousand samples were collected from the Dry Tortugas for serological and virological study.

Four years later we mounted an expedition to the Guano Islands. It was supported by the WHO in conjunction with the Peruvian government, which supplied its research ship for transport to the islands. We collected thousands of serum samples, throat swabs and faecal samples from these huge populations of birds, which spend their entire lives at sea except when they nest and raise their young. Both studies came up empty in that we detected no antibodies or influenza viruses in any of the samples. Clearly not all populations of pelagic birds were infected with influenza. Finding those that were would require being at the right place at the right time. We needed to change our approach.

I decided to focus on my own back yard. Publications from colleagues had reported the detection of antibodies to avian influenza viruses in migratory Canadian geese (*Branta canadensis*),[30] and influenza viruses had been found in free-flying ducks in California.[31] Since Memphis lies on the Mississippi Flyway, the route taken by migratory waterfowl flying from Canada to their overwintering grounds in South America, it is an excellent site for studying these birds.

Each year millions of wild ducks and geese fly south, and each year hunters harvest a portion of them. The numbers of ducks and geese that hunters can shoot and the length of the hunting season in different areas are set by the Canadian and American wildlife authorities, who monitor the bird populations. Hunting is usually permitted in two periods: one in mid- to late November and the other in early December.

Obtaining samples from waterfowl shot by hunters turned out to be easy. Many American hunters don't like to dress (clean) their own ducks, so they take them to a dressing station, where they pay to have them gutted and plucked. With the permission of the owner of the Minnow Bucket, a dressing station in West Memphis, Arkansas, we joined two very cheerful women in the back room to collect samples from the ducks before they were dressed. The employees held the dead ducks against a rotating drum with long rubber fingers that removed all of the down and feathers. They then eviscerated and washed the ducks and gave them back to the hunters beautifully wrapped and ready for cooking. The feathers were bagged for marketing to down and feather bedding and clothing manufacturers. Meanwhile we collected throat swabs from the ducks and stored them in a chilly bin (cooler) containing ice.

Back in the laboratory, a small volume of the solution surrounding the swab was injected into 10-day-old developing chicken eggs, as described in Chapter 2. The eggs were kept for two days at 35°C, and then a small sample of fluid was removed to test for the presence of virus by adding a few drops of chicken red blood cells. If an influenza virus was present, the cells would clump or haemagglutinate.

In the very first batch of samples from the ducks we found influenza virus, which was designated A/Duck/Memphis/546/74 (H11N9). Like the influenza virus from birds on the Great Barrier Reef, this virus caused no disease when put into the throat and eyes of young ducks.[32]

In that first season of sampling wild ducks, approximately 2 per cent of the birds yielded influenza viruses of different subtypes. We wanted to know if the virus had increased to high levels in the ducks and whether it was present anywhere besides the respiratory tract. A visiting Russian scientist, Maya Yakhno, was given the job of separating all of the organs from the infected ducks and determining the level of virus in each. This simple study resulted in another of those eureka moments. Yakhno found that the virus was present in all parts of the intestinal tract she examined, and that the highest amount of virus was in the faeces. This finding eventually led to the significant realisation that in aquatic birds, the influenza virus caused an intestinal infection.[33] Virus counts in the faeces were as high as 100 million virus units per gram of faeces. The virus was probably spread from bird to bird through contaminated water. This meant that hunters could easily tramp influenza viruses on their boots back to their homes – and, if they were farmers, to their poultry houses. It also meant that wild ducks could contaminate smaller ponds with enough viruses to infect other animals.

Since Memphis is well along in the birds' southern migration route, we wondered if the incidence we detected was low because we were detecting the end of an outbreak. Perhaps the best place to look for influenza in wild ducks would be in Canada during the summer, when the wildlife authorities banded birds for identification before their migration south. I sent out about 20 letters to Canadian wildlife officials explaining the proposed study. I received a reply from Bruce Turner of the Edmonton office of the Canadian Wildlife Service (now part of Environment Canada), who agreed to let me join his banding team in July 1976. I flew to Edmonton with the same array of equipment that we had used on the Great Barrier Reef – Dacron throat swabs, collection vials, vials for serum and a Dewar flask of liquid nitrogen for cold storage of the samples (Figure 4.1).

Turner's banding team was an extremely cooperative group of young men who made me very welcome. Their trucks were loaded with duck traps and bags of grain. These traps were large wire cages that birds could swim into but not get out of. The traps were baited with grain and set on floating polystyrene blocks near the edges of the small lakes in southern Alberta, near Vermillion. A hessian grain bag over the trap protected the captive ducks from getting too much sun.

The next morning each trap contained five to ten birds. The species of each bird was recorded (mallard, pintail, etc.) before the bird was given a leg band with a unique number and its age was assessed. Young ducks grow so quickly that it took an expert to decide whether they were juveniles or adults. Very occasionally a bird already had a band; this information was recorded, and the bird was given a second band.

I took swab samples initially just from the throat, but by the second year, as at the Great Barrier Reef, I sampled both ends of the bird, as well as collecting a blood sample from the wing vein. The men bringing the ducks ashore were very patient – the swabbing and bleeding slowed down their normal banding work and made some days very long. All ducks, of all the different species, were fat and healthy, preparing for their southern migration.

Turner and his crew were very sceptical that any of these healthy birds could possibly carry the influenza virus. We discussed the matter many evenings over dinner, since they were all biologists and not easily put off their food! I was left with the distinct impression that they were tolerating a rather nutty professor determined to take butt swabs from robust birds.

But analysis of the samples in the Memphis laboratory yielded amazing results: up to 18.5 per cent of juvenile birds (hatched that year) and 5 per cent of adults were excreting influenza viruses. While one strain of influenza was dominant, small numbers of many different subtypes were isolated.[34] When the results were sent back to Turner and his crew, I hope they decided the professor wasn't so nutty after all (Figure 4.2).

This sampling of wild ducks in Canada has been going on for nearly 40 years now, and not all the outcomes are published in the scientific literature or followed up. One sampling study attempted to determine whether the fish in the lakes are infected with influenza from the ducks or contain detectable levels of virus. In the second year of sampling (1977), I had driven from Memphis to Alberta with my family with the usual sampling supplies but also had a gill net for catching fish, specially made by the North American department store Sears Roebuck.

At the first sampling site on the first morning. I rolled out the gill net from my car and asked Turner where I should put it. Turner was a Newfoundlander and unfazed by most things. On this occasion, however, he went bright purple and told me exactly where I should put that net. I didn't know that gill nets were illegal in Canada or that for wildlife personnel to be seen with one would be scandalous. No fish were sampled for influenza on that trip.

That night my youngest son, James, surprised everyone by catching his limit of very large northern pike (*Esox lucius*) on a 10-cent white woolly lure that he had bought in Memphis at a variety store. The

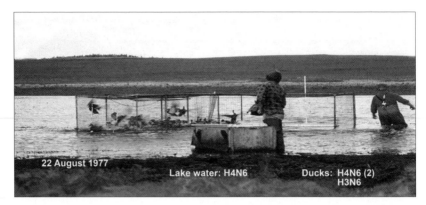

22 August 1977

Lake water: H4N6

Ducks: H4N6 (2)
H3N6

Figure 4.1 A duck trap on a lake near Vermillion, Alberta, Canada, with Bruce Turner (red shirt) of the Canadian Wildlife Services (now part of Environment Canada) showing the different influenza viruses isolated from the ducks in the trap and the water, on 22 August 1977.

locals, who were not getting bites, came to inspect his lure. In our eagerness to eat the catch, we forgot to sample the fish before cooking them, so despite over 40 years of collaborative study on influenza with Canadian wildlife personnel, I have still never taken scientific samples from the fish.

On the return road trip to Memphis after that sampling trip, my wife Marjorie was the driver, taking the family and the samples back to Memphis, the latter in the insulated liquid nitrogen container. I had flown to Australia to join Laver. As my family headed south that morning, the children wanted to know why that car behind had all those flashing lights. Marjorie's first worry was the samples – and whether she had copies of the right import permits. The police officer was very gracious about her travelling over 80 miles per hour when he saw that the car was registered in Tennessee. He asked if she was hurrying back for Elvis Presley's funeral, which was to take place the next day. He then asked her to slow down, for at the time the speed limit on United States highways was 55 miles per hour.

Subtypes	N1	N2	N3	N4	N5	N6	N7	N8	N9	TOTALS
H1	145	15	7	0	3	5	0	2	1	178
H2	1	1	28	4	2	0	0	0	5	41
H3	34	23	4	3	10	94	0	1038	6	1215
H4	5	46	6	8	9	673	0	50	4	801
H5	0	6	1	0	1	0	0	0	0	8
H6	7	718	5	13	167	167	0	110	4	1191
H7	3	1	32	0	0	0	0	6	2	44
H8	0	0	0	15	0	0	0	0	0	15
H9	6	5	0	0	3	1	0	0	0	15
H10	3	0	1	1	1	4	52	1	0	63
H11	0	1	1	1	2	2	0	1	31	39
H12	2	0	0	1	22	0	0	1	0	26
H13	0	0	0	0	0	0	0	0	0	0
H14	0	0	0	0	0	0	0	0	0	0
H15	0	0	0	0	0	0	0	0	0	0
H16	0	0	0	0	0	0	0	0	0	0
TOTALS	206	816	85	46	220	946	52	1209	56	3636

All low pathogenic

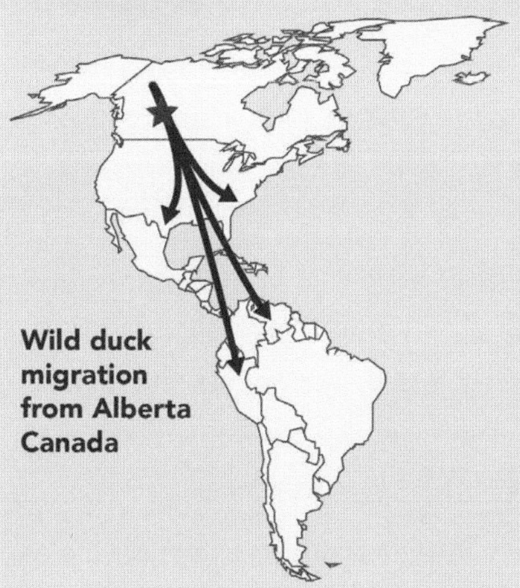

Wild duck migration from Alberta Canada

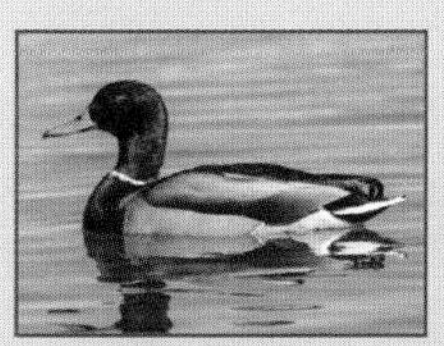

Mallard

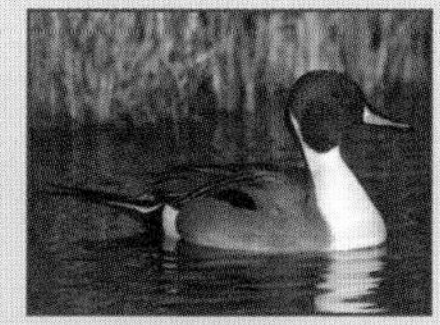

Pintail

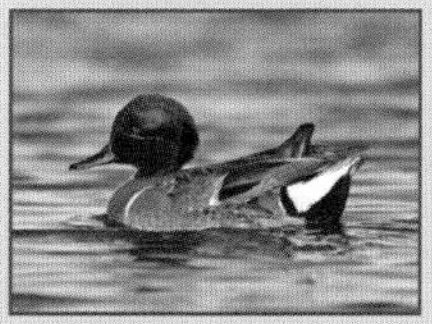

Green wing teal

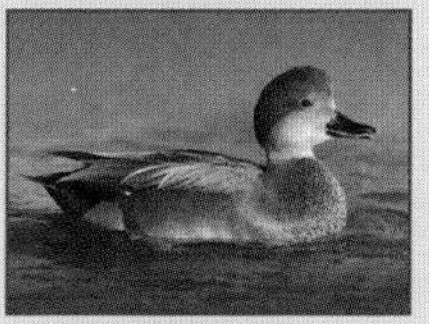

Gadwall

Figure 4.2 Results of surveillance for influenza viruses among wild ducks in Alberta, Canada, 1976–2016, showing the different combinations of haemagglutinin and neuraminidase. The dominant viruses change from year to year, with H1N1, H3N8, H4N6, H6N2, H6N5 and H6N6 the most frequently isolated viruses. Counterparts of human H1N1 and H3N2 were isolated, but H2N2 was isolated only once. No isolates of H13, H14, H15 and H16 were detected in these migratory ducks. Several different duck species were sampled, including mallard, pintail, gadwall and teal, and the dominant influenza virus was isolated from all species. Most duck species migrate to the southern states of United States to overwinter, but the teals migrate as far as northern South America. Table courtesy of Scott Krauss, St Jude Children's Research Hospital

The other question that remained unanswered was whether influenza viruses overwinter in the frozen lakes and re-infect the ducks when they return in the spring. In midwinter 1978 Turner and his team drilled holes in the ice and sampled the water. We never did succeed in isolating influenza viruses from the dozens of water samples, but other studies showed that in the laboratory these viruses remain viable for months at low temperatures. Later, in the collaborative studies, our Canadian colleagues collected cloacal and throat swabs from ducks on their northern spring migration returning to their breeding grounds in Canada. Approximately 0.2 per cent of the apparently healthy returning ducks were 'shedding' influenza viruses of different subtypes. Thus it is possible that the influenza viruses remain present in a flock over winter, albeit at low levels, but we cannot rule out the possibility that some influenza viruses come from the lakes after thawing.

* * *

Initial scepticism towards our findings gave way to acceptance. Our pioneering studies of Canadian ducks in many ways triggered the global interest in influenza viruses in aquatic birds and established many of the now-accepted ecological principles of influenza viruses, including the fact that wild aquatic birds are indeed a major reservoir of the influenza viruses that evolve into pandemic viruses for humans. The studies continue to the present day. In 1975 the WHO invited St Jude Children's Research Hospital to become a collaborating centre on the Ecology of Influenza Viruses at the human–animal interface, a role it continues to fulfil.

CHAPTER 5

DELAWARE BAY: THE RIGHT PLACE AT THE RIGHT TIME

One of the most significant natural events in the ecology of influenza viruses occurs each May on the beaches of Delaware Bay, New Jersey. Tens of thousands of horseshoe crabs come ashore on the first full moon in May to mate and lay their eggs in the sand. At just this time, migrating shorebirds (red knots and ruddy turnstones) are arriving in their tens of thousands, having flown non-stop from South America. The migration of these birds is timed so that they can refuel on horseshoe crab eggs, gaining up to 30 per cent of their body weight before setting out on the next flight, to Churchill Bay in Canada, en route to the far north of Canada, where they in turn mate and breed. In Delaware Bay, the birds deliver influenza viruses to beaches that are shared with the resident gulls and wading birds that also feed on horseshoe crab eggs.[35] The horseshoe crab is known as the 'keynote species' in this amazing sequence of events.[36]

The horseshoe crab (*Limulus polyphemus*) is an extremely ancient creature, having evolved even before dinosaurs. It lives on the floor of oceans and bays, feeding on worms and other invertebrates. These crabs can be found on the beaches of the east coast of North America from Maine to Mexico, but by far the highest population density occurs at Delaware Bay.

At the first full moon in May, the male crabs arrive. The females, nearly twice the size of the males, arrive soon after. The male selects a mate and attaches himself to her with a special limb. The female digs holes in the wet sand and deposits her eggs in them for the attached male – and additional unattached males – to fertilise. Each female may lay as many as five nests of eggs – up to 80,000 eggs in all.

In the 1980s the beaches at Delaware Bay were covered with horseshoe crabs, and the waterline was marked by a layer of green crab eggs washed from the sand.

These eggs are just the fuel that the migratory shorebirds need after their four-day flight from Lagoa de Peixe National Park in southern Brazil (a distance of 4828 kilometres). Up to 25 species of seabird converge on Delaware Bay in May to feast on horseshoe crab eggs.[37] In addition to the red knot (*Calidris canutus*) and the ruddy turnstone (*Arenaria interpres*), the most abundant are the sanderling (*Calidris alba*), the semi-palmated sandpiper (*Calidris pusilla*) and three species of gull: the great black-backed gull (*Larus marinus*), herring gull (*Larus argentatus*) and laughing gull (*Leucophaeus atricilla*). The most amazing are the red knots, which migrate from Tierra del Fuego, at the tip of South America, in three hops to Delaware Bay (Figure 5.1). Before this long-distance migration they gorge themselves, consuming up to 14 times their body weight in mussel sprats and converting them to fat. At that point, the physiology of the bird changes: those organs not needed for flight (the liver, leg muscles and gut) shrivel in size to accommodate more stored fat. This means the birds cannot digest solid food en route; the gelatinous horseshoe crab eggs at Delaware Bay are the perfect fare.

The shorebird that turned out to be of most interest from our perspective was the ruddy turnstone. These birds (and the other species) arrive from the Atlantic east coast of the United States and from the northern coast of South America, often having joined red knots on the final leg of their migration. The two species compete for

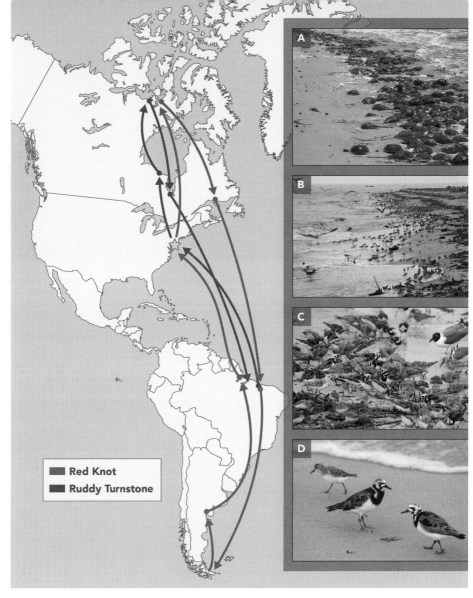

Figure 5.1 The migration routes of red knots and ruddy turnstones. The red knots travel in three hops from Tierra del Fuego, at the tip of South America, to Delaware Bay, and from there head to northern Canada to breed. The ruddy turnstones join the migration from the north of South America. Some turnstones follow the coastline to Delaware Bay. At the first full moon in May the horseshoe crabs come ashore at Delaware Bay (gold star) to lay their eggs in the sand (A). The resident gulls and shorebirds (B) are joined by red knots and ruddy turnstones (C, D) which have migrated long distances to refuel on the horseshoe crab eggs. The ruddy turnstone, the bird of greatest interest, is shown separately in D, while panel C shows a mixture of mainly red knots and ruddy turnstones. The leg band on the ruddy turnstone (D) was added during the annual counting and swabbing of the birds. Photos courtesy of Jere Parobek, St Jude Children's Reasearch Hospital

food on the way to their breeding grounds in the Canadian Arctic.

Since our two attempts to detect influenza viruses in American seabirds (Guano Islands, Peru; Dry Tortugas, Florida) had not been fruitful, our team from St Jude Children's Research Hospital was looking for the right time and place to try again. Research results presented at a scientific meeting in 1983 by Larry Graves about the detection of several influenza viruses in gulls at a Baltimore landfill in 1977–79 provided the first clue. The written report appeared many years later.[38] The next clue came from an English ornithologist, William (Bill) Slayden, who was aware of the Delaware Bay shorebird migration in May and suggested sampling at that time.

On the first visit to Delaware Bay, in May 1985, we went on our own and with no idea where to find the birds. We eventually found them at Reeds Beach. The sight was quite amazing: the beach was littered with overturned horseshoe crab shells and packed with shorebirds in a feeding frenzy as they dug in the wet sand for crab eggs. As some birds left, more came in. Most were red knots and ruddy turnstones. The collection of fresh faecal samples was easy. We followed the birds along the waterline, collecting freshly deposited droppings on a Dacron swab and putting them into vials containing 50 per cent glycerol with antibiotics to suppress bacterial growth. The collection vials went directly into a cooler containing ordinary ice blocks. Within three days of collection, the samples were air-freighted to the laboratory in Memphis.

There, additional antibiotic was added to each sample and a small amount of the total was injected into 10-day-old developing chicken eggs and held for two days at 35°C. The very first tray of eggs yielded many samples that agglutinated chicken red blood cells, indicating that an influenza or parainfluenza virus was present. (A parainfluenza virus is a virus that comes from wild birds and can infect and kill chickens.) Some 20 per cent of the samples tested positive for influenza viruses.[39] We were ecstatic. In the following two years, we isolated influenza viruses belonging to 10 of the 12 different haemagglutinin (H) subtypes of influenza viruses known at that time. These included influenza viruses of the H1N1 group, related to the virus that caused the 1918 Spanish influenza pandemic, and the H3N2 group, responsible for the 1968 Hong Kong pandemic. We also found viruses belonging to the H7N3 subtype, which can evolve into lethal influenza in chickens and turkeys.

We realised that we had stumbled on a goldmine of influenza viruses, and we have mined that source every year since. Most of the viruses came from ruddy turnstones. Sampling of the resident gulls, sanderlings, terns and other shorebirds at monthly intervals over three years detected high levels of influenza virus in May and June but very low levels in September and October; there were no detectable viruses in other months. The small incidence in September and October may come from occasional arrivals by red knots and ruddy turnstones on their return migration. The zero readings in other months illustrate why single-shot sampling of waterfowl can fail to isolate viruses. It really is a case of being in the right place at the right time.

After our findings, influenza virologists in Europe, Asia and Australia began sampling the same species in their countries. They did find influenza viruses, but the incidence was much lower than what we found in May and June in Delaware Bay. Some of our international colleagues found it hard to believe our results and even came to Delaware Bay on the quiet to test for themselves. They confirmed our results.

We now know that Delaware Bay is a hotspot for influenza viruses during migration of the red knots and other shorebirds,[40] but we still don't know why. We can speculate that the migrating birds are stressed after their long migration and therefore may be susceptible to infection. The ruddy turnstones arriving from coastal regions of the United States have no detectable antibodies to any influenza viruses, and the huge congregations of these birds with other species provide optimal conditions for influenza to spread. But what is the actual source of the viruses? One possibility is that the ruddy turnstones, which are voracious scavengers, pick up viruses from other animals or birds or even human waste from the coastal towns of northern South America.[41] But we don't know for sure, showing that there are still important mysteries to solve.

Over the years, many volunteers have helped collect samples at Delaware Bay, including researchers' granddaughters. One of mine, at the age of three, helpfully pointed out, 'Look, Grandad, bird poop!' Other helpers have included National Geographic documentary crews who have documented influenza surveillance at Delaware Bay. Senior molecular biologists who visit cannot believe that these beautiful, healthy birds, which have flown all the way from South America, could be carrying influenza viruses.

From our 30-plus years of surveying influenza viruses at Delaware Bay, we have assembled a huge collection of influenza viruses. Currently, there are 16 subtypes of influenza A virus identified from aquatic birds in nature. Fifteen of these subtypes are found in both ducks and shorebirds. H15 has not been found in the Americas to date but has been found in Eurasian waterfowl.

The different subtypes have different cycles of dominance. One subtype will dominate for one year in one region and be replaced by another subtype the next year. These viruses from ducks and shorebirds provided the background information that enabled us to propose in the late 1990s the following ecological principles of the ecology of influenza A viruses:

- Wild aquatic birds are the natural reservoirs of most of the influenza A viruses found in other species (including humans) (Figure 5.2). Two subtypes of influenza virus have recently been found in bats, so there is more work to be done on identifying virus reservoirs.

Subtypes	N1	N2	N3	N4	N5	N6	N7	N8	N9	TOTALS
H1	30	5	10	8	2	1	3	7	39	105
H2	10	0	3	2	0	0	6	3	3	27
H3	5	44	4	7	3	34	1	72	0	170
H4	0	0	0	0	0	52	0	1	9	62
H5	5	7	4	8	0	0	2	7	4	37
H6	11	15	1	15	2	0	0	31	1	76
H7	3	2	74	5	2	0	8	2	1	97
H8	0	0	0	3	0	0	0	0	0	3
H9	5	26	0	9	21	2	5	5	22	95
H10	14	15	0	13	29	2	109	16	8	206
H11	12	47	4	19	0	1	10	6	68	167
H12	2	3	8	55	59	0	14	2	3	146
H13	1	20	2	1	0	29	1	0	3	57
H14	0	0	0	0	0	0	0	0	0	0
H15	0	0	0	0	0	0	0	0	0	0
H16	0	1	14	0	0	4	0	0	0	19
TOTALS	98	185	124	145	118	125	159	152	161	1267

All low pathogenic

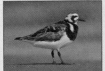

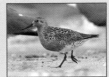

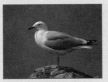

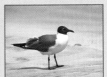

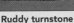

| **Ruddy turnstone** | **Red knot** | **Herring gull** | **Laughing gull** |

Figure 5.2 Results of surveillance for influenza viruses among shorebirds and gulls at Delaware Bay, 1985–2016. As in migratory ducks, the dominant viruses changed from year to year. A wide variety of combinations was isolated, including counterparts of human H1N1 and H3N2, but no H2N2 was detected. It is noteworthy that the H7N3 virus was isolated quite frequently and was the precursor of influenza viruses that became killer strains in domestic poultry in Chile and Mexico. No H14 or H15 viruses were isolated, but H13 and H16 viruses not detected in Alberta wild ducks were present in these shorebirds and gulls. Table courtesy of Scott Krauss, St Jude Children's Research Hospital

- The viruses replicate predominantly in the intestinal tracts of aquatic birds.

- They cause no apparent disease signs and are considered 'low-pathogenic'.

- There is geographical separation into Eurasian and American lineages.

- Two subtypes, H5 and H7, are unique and can become highly pathogenic after they spread to domestic chickens and turkeys.

- Only the H1, H2 and H3 subtypes are known to have caused pandemics of influenza in humans.

For many years some of these conclusions were treated with considerable scepticism, especially the idea that human pandemics could emerge from aquatic birds. This changed after the emergence of the H5N1 virus, dubbed 'bird flu', in Hong Kong in 1997. Since then there has been gradual acceptance of the 'one world, one health' concept that viruses that are benign in non-human animal reservoirs – such as influenza, Zika and SARS (severe acute respiratory syndrome) – can become killers when they spread to other animals, including humans (Figure 5.3).

ONE WORLD, ONE HEALTH

The one world, one health concept is based on the realisation that the health of humans and animals (domestic and wild) is intimately linked to the ecosystems in which they live. As many as 60 per cent of known human diseases originate from domestic or wild animals and birds. Influenza is one of the diseases that exemplifies this concept.

Before 1980, influenza viruses were divided into four separate groups according to the species they were believed to infect: one for humans, one for swine, one for equines and one for avians. But after influenza scientists recognised that influenza viruses from different species were intimately interconnected, a uniform nomenclature system was developed in 1980.

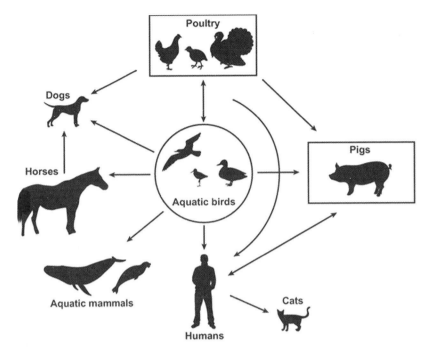

Figure 5.3 A diagram showing the natural reservoirs of influenza A viruses in wild aquatic birds (in the circle) and transmission through intermediate hosts to mammals including humans. The solid black lines indicate possible inter-species transmission. The boxes indicate the species that serve as intermediate hosts and are most likely involved in the emergence of zoonotic viruses with pandemic potential. (Influenza viruses have been isolated from bats but their role in interspecies transmission is not known.)

The huge abundance of horseshoe crabs led to their exploitation by humans in the mid-twentieth century. Since they contain little edible tissue, they were ground up for agricultural fertiliser and chicken food. Because the crabs exude a strong attractant odour when cut into sections, they were also used as bait by conch and eel fishermen.

The horseshoe crab has also contributed to our understanding of human vision. The crab has a huge optic nerve that allowed Haldan Keffer Hartline to explain how the receptors in the eye enable us to see. His research led to his receiving the 1967 Nobel Prize in Physiology and Medicine (jointly with Ragnar Gramit and George Wald).

In addition, studies on the blood of the horseshoe crab have identified a particular component that protects the crab from infection in its murky environment. The component, known as limulus amebocyte lysate (LAL), is extracted to form the basis for a clinical test for bacterial endotoxin contamination (a toxin produced in a bacterial cell that can cause disease symptoms in humans). This test is now required by the United States Food and Drug Administration for testing of all instruments, drugs and vaccines (including the influenza vaccine) for biological contamination, and it is also used in Europe and Japan. Consequently up to 250,000 crabs are caught each year and blood samples collected for the LAL preparation by pharmaceutical firms. The crabs are returned to Delaware Bay after the procedure, but 15–30 per cent of them die.[42]

Unsurprisingly, these human uses of horseshoe crabs have led to their severe depletion. Grinding the crabs up for fertiliser ended after cheaper artificial fertilisers became available, but the demand by conch and eel fishermen increased. By the 1990s the crab population had dropped tenfold or more, with disastrous effects on the migratory shorebirds that feed on the crab eggs. The numbers of red knots and ruddy turnstones fell by 86 and 75 per cent respectively. Many birds failed to gain the threshold weight they needed for the Arctic flight and perished on their trip to their Arctic breeding grounds. By 2006 the numbers of red knots had fallen by another 86 per cent from their 1980s level.

However, thanks to coastal conservation and resource management efforts by the American Littoral Society and the Atlantic States Marine Fish Commission, the harvesting of horseshoe crabs is now banned between 1 May and 7 June. Each state has capped the harvest at 150,000, and conch fishermen are required to use bait-saving devices like bait bags, reducing crab use. Beach access by humans is restricted in late May.

Once horseshoe crabs are flipped onto their backs they have great difficulty turning back over, which is one reason the beaches were littered with crab shells on our first visits. Many of our visiting colleagues and family members spend most of their time turning the crabs right side up again so they can make it back to the sea. This rescue of horseshoe crabs is vital.

The numbers of red knots stabilised and now are gradually increasing, but the numbers of ruddy turnstones remain low. Neither the frequency nor the diversity of influenza viruses has changed with the decline in migrating shorebirds, but collecting samples is more difficult. Influenza virologists work closely with the conservation agencies protecting the birds to ensure minimal disturbance of feeding birds while collecting faecal samples from the beaches, and when the birds are caught by wildlife experts for banding in population studies, virologists take the opportunity to collect samples at the same time.

CHAPTER 6

PROVING INTERSPECIES TRANSMISSION

Back in the 1960s, after the emergence of the devastating Asian H2N2 influenza virus, I started contacting people who stored influenza viruses. I wanted to determine if any of these viruses might be related to the pandemic-causing strain that had killed at least 1.5 million people in 1957. One of the largest collections of influenza viruses – from humans, horses, pigs and birds – was in Helio Pereira's laboratory at the National Institute of Medical Research in Mill Hill, London.

Pereira was the director of the World Influenza Centre, which was one of the World Health Organization (WHO) laboratories collaborating on influenza research, and he, like me, was a proponent of the animal reservoir hypothesis to explain the origin of human influenza pandemics. He was very interested to know whether we could find any cross-reactivity between the recently identified Asian H2N2 influenza viruses and other influenza viruses from various animals in his collection. Běla Tůmová, an influenza virologist from Czechoslovakia who had made antisera in rats to the H2N2 virus and to some of the animal influenza viruses, joined the study.[43] Antisera contain virus-specific antibodies made by the body in response to infection or vaccination; antisera are used to identify unknown influenza viruses.

In the initial study in 1967 we used the rat sera from Czechoslovakia and ferret sera from Mill Hill to determine whether any of the sera to the animal influenza viruses would react with the human influenza virus. We found in three quite different tests that there was a strong reaction between an influenza virus isolated from turkeys in Massachusetts in 1965 and the human influenza virus that had caused the 1957 pandemic. The reaction was so strong that we did not quite believe the results and worried that somehow the human viruses had been contaminated with animal ones or vice versa. Exhaustive studies ruled out that possibility, and we concluded that indeed we had found that the turkey and human influenza viruses had something in common. We were absolutely delighted, for this provided some of the first solid evidence supporting the hypothesis that animal influenza viruses are the source of at least part of the pandemic influenza viruses. Our next step was to determine which part of the turkey and human influenza viruses was shared – the neuraminidase (N) spike, as we thought, or the haemagglutinin (H).[44]

While these studies were under way in London, my close colleague Graeme Laver in Canberra had successfully separated the two major surface spikes on influenza virus – the haemagglutinin (H) and the neuraminidase (N) – in chemically pure forms. On my return to Canberra I prepared antisera in rabbits to the pure H and pure N components and showed that we could specifically identify each of them. Pereira encouraged me to bring these antisera to London to answer the question of which components were shared by the turkey virus and human pandemic virus.

In a whirlwind two-day trip back to Mill Hill in early 1967 we set up the neuraminidase inhibition test used in the Great Barrier Reef studies and showed that the specific antisera to neuraminidase from the 1957 influenza virus completely inhibited the enzyme activity of the turkey influenza virus. We also found that three other avian influenza viruses in Pereira's virus collection possessed a neuraminidase very closely related to, or serologically identical with, the neuraminidase of the human 1957 influenza virus. One of these viruses was obtained from turkeys in Wisconsin in 1966, and two were obtained from ducks in Italy in the same year.[45] These findings further supported the idea that the human pandemic influenza virus of 1957 had acquired its neuraminidase component from an animal influenza virus.

But was it possible for human influenza viruses to acquire pieces of animal influenza viruses under natural conditions? I knew of the early studies by Frank Macfarlane Burnet and Patricia Lind in Melbourne, who had put two different influenza A viruses into chicken embryos together and found that the viruses reassorted (exchanged) their genome segments, resulting in hybrid viruses.[46] If we did a similar experiment using chickens and pigs, we too might generate new influenza viruses. But because the hybrids might be dangerous to pigs or poultry, this research required a highly secure environment. Since we had no high-containment laboratories at St Jude Children's Research Hospital in Memphis in 1970, I approached the agricultural authorities at the high-containment laboratories on Plum Island, off the northwest end of Long Island, New York.

The laboratories at Plum Island are designed to protect American livestock from 'exotic' animal diseases and their causal agents. By studying such exotic agents under high-security conditions, the scientists develop vaccines, antiviral agents and control strategies in case these agents are ever introduced into the country. Jerry Callis, the director of the Plum Island facility, was extremely interested in my proposal. Fowl plague can kill every chicken, turkey or other type of poultry that contracts it (see Chapter 2), and Plum Island had no scientists working on this enormous potential threat to the American poultry industry. Callis invited me to visit the island and present the proposed study to his staff. The staff were also positive, and Charles

Campbell agreed to provide space and training so that my colleague Allen Granoff and I could work in his high-security laboratories.

Since Plum Island is approximately 2000 kilometres from Memphis, and these experiments were going to take several weeks to complete, it was necessary to organise travel and accommodation. Travel was straightforward: by air to New York, then by bus to Greenport, Long Island, the nearest small town to Plum Island, and then by private government ferry to the island itself. For the last leg, we needed either to have a security pass or to be travelling with a security-cleared staff member.

Once we had settled in, we realised that the cost of our mainland accommodation was quickly going to become prohibitive. Charles Campbell, my adopted mentor at Plum Island, came to the rescue and asked Callis if we could stay in the safety officer's accommodation on the island. (One senior scientific officer always stayed on the island every night in case storms prevented the ferry from bringing staff to care for the experimental animals.) Callis agreed, and the arrangement was a tremendous bonus. Although we had to prepare our own meals and clean our rooms, we also had uninterrupted time to discuss science with the safety officer.

Turning up for work each day at the laboratories entailed disrobing and donning clothes to be worn on site only. At the end of the workday we had to leave all work clothing behind, take a thorough shower and put on street clothes. Nothing but people left the laboratories. All the air from the building was filtered to remove any particulate material, including viruses, and all water and waste were autoclaved. Once they were approved as completely sterile, they were discarded into the sea.

In the first experiment, Granoff and I investigated whether two different avian influenza viruses would exchange their haemagglutinin (H) and neuraminidase (N) surface spikes when they were put into a turkey together. Since these experiments were done in the era before genome sequencing became readily available, the only way to identify the H and N protein components on the viruses was with the specific antibodies used in the studies with Pereira.[47] The turkeys were infected with the killer fowl plague virus (H7N7) and the turkey influenza virus (H6N2). The latter, which caused mild disease in poultry, shared its neuraminidase (N2) with the virus of the 1957 human influenza pandemic. The turkeys began to die after two days, and we found that one in every four viruses from the respiratory tract had reassorted their H and N proteins to produce H7N2 and H6N7 hybrid viruses. The H7N2 viruses were lethal to turkeys.[48]

In the second experiment, pigs were co-infected with two influenza viruses, one that could multiply in pigs and one that did not. For the former, we used the classical H1N1 swine influenza virus, the descendant of 1918 Spanish influenza virus that persisted in pigs. For the latter, we used the fowl plague virus. Two days later the pigs had a high fever of 40°C, and in lung samples we found that some of the viruses present had exchanged their H and N surface spikes (Figure 6.1).

In both experiments we found fewer reassorted viruses than parent ones, and the novel hybrid viruses were detected only after we had suppressed the parental viruses with antiserum specific to them. This led us to ask whether selection in nature could result in such new viruses becoming dominant. So, in the next experiments, we put our various infected turkeys in contact with birds vaccinated with the influenza viruses found in nature, with the expectation that the vaccine would suppress the parent viruses. Influenza viruses possessing the H7 protein of the fowl plague virus and the turkey virus N2 protein were detected in the vaccinated contact birds and rapidly killed them.

In the pig version of these experiments, we decided to use the human H3N2 influenza A virus, which had spread to pigs and then been re-isolated from pigs, and the classical H1N1 swine influenza

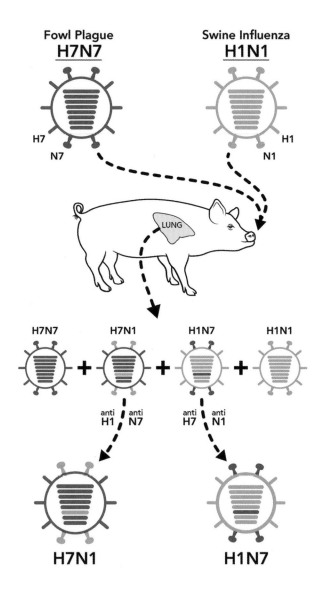

Figure 6.1 Reassortment of influenza viruses in pigs. Pigs were given, in the nose, a mixture of fowl plague H7N7 influenza virus (which did not multiply in the pig) and swine influenza H1N1 influenza (which did multiply). Two days later the pigs had a high fever (40°C) and were euthanased. Their lungs contained numerous influenza viruses, including the parental pair, H7N7 and H1N1, and the hybrid viruses H7N1 and H1N7. The hybrid influenza viruses were isolated by growing the mixed viruses from the lungs in the presence of antibodies specific for H7 plus N1, or H1 plus N7.

virus. However, this time we made the experiment more like a real-world situation by putting one virus into one pig and the second virus into another pig. After six hours, both pigs were introduced into a group of four contact non-vaccinated pigs. By the seventh day we detected H3N1 hybrid influenza viruses (with the H3 haemagglutinin from the human virus and the N1 neuraminidase from the swine virus) and the other possible hybrid virus (H1N2) in one of the four contact pigs.

These experiments showed that when influenza viruses from different species co-infect an animal, new hybrid influenza viruses can emerge. Thus, the N2 on the virus that caused the 1957 human pandemic could have been a hybrid that emerged from animals.

The results from all these experiments were very exciting, and everyone in Campbell's laboratory at Plum Island realised that we had hit a home run. Influenza viruses in different animals could indeed mix and exchange components under natural conditions, and the resultant hybrids could become dominant.

There was one drama while we were there that was a bit too exciting. During the second series of experiments with pigs and human influenza viruses in 1972, the laboratory technologist holding the animals called in sick two days after the experiment had started. The next day he phoned to say that he was severely ill, with a high fever. We were very concerned. While we had ensured the protection of the animal population and the environment, the protection measures for humans were rather primitive. We wore gloves, masks and gowns, and we had our showering routine, but we lacked the kind of personal protective equipment that would be required for such experiments today, such as a powered air-purifying respirator (PAPR) with a hood and mask, which covers the face entirely.

On the third day the technologist left a message to say he had been diagnosed with mumps, and there was a collective sigh of relief.

(Though of course mumps can be a serious infection for an adult male, he recovered with no long-term consequences.) Although the incident did not result in human transmission, it made us aware of how easily influenza viruses could be spread between animals and then exchange components. I was convinced that it would be only a matter of time before we found evidence for this reassortment in the natural world. In fact we did not find it for nearly three decades, until the H5N1 bird flu outbreaks in Hong Kong in 1997 (see Chapters 10 and 11).

In tandem with the reassortment investigations outlined above, we began to look for possible parent or precursor viruses for the H3N2 Hong Kong influenza pandemic of 1968. Since only the H spike of this virus was new, we focused on this spike in our search. Through WHO collaborations we obtained influenza viruses from ducks, pigs and horses from around the world to compare with the H3N2 virus. Two viruses of interest emerged from our comparisons. An influenza virus isolated from horses in Miami in 1963 had a similar H spike to that on H3N2, as did one from ducks in the Ukraine obtained that same year.[49]

To determine the extent of molecular similarity among the three haemagglutinin proteins, in 1972 Laver isolated the haemagglutinin from all the viruses and 'mapped' their peptides. Peptide mapping was a key method of studying proteins before the age of sequence analysis. It produces a map of the peptides (short sequences of amino acids) that make up a protein. Identical proteins have maps that completely overlay each other. If the proteins are completely different, their maps do not coincide at all; if they are slightly different, a few spots do not coincide.

Part of the haemagglutinin of the duck, horse and human influenza viruses was identical (the backbone light chain), while the rest of the molecule had a small number of differences, according to the peptide maps.[50] These molecular studies explained the similarities we and others had found among sera targeting isolated H spikes, and they added to an increasing body of evidence from studies on the virus of

Asian 1957 H2N2 and the virus of Hong Kong 1968 H3N2 that animal influenza viruses contribute component parts of pandemic influenza viruses.

I learned one of life's unforgettable lessons after my whirlwind visit to Pereira's laboratory at Mill Hill to set up the neuraminidase inhibition test to identify which component turkey and human influenza viruses shared. The final test results came out very close to my plane's departure time, and in the rush to catch the plane, I put all of the data from the experiments in my checked baggage. On arrival in Hong Kong, my luggage was missing, and I became frantic because we had no copy of the data (this was 1967, before the computer age). The airline was very helpful, but it took over an hour to locate my suitcase, languishing at Heathrow because of my late check-in. It was put on a later flight to Hong Kong, and I was very relieved to receive it before boarding my flight to Canberra.

Another life lesson followed shortly thereafter. One of the greatest disappointments for a scientist is to have work that he or she considers earth-shaking rejected for publication by a scientific journal. This is what happened to us with the Plum Island studies. My colleagues at Plum Island and at St Jude were excited about the results, which showed for the first time that influenza viruses 'in a real-world situation', when the right conditions were present, could easily reassort their genes and produce a new or novel virus. I was the most excited, for the findings offered a possible explanation for the genesis of both the Asian 1957 and Hong Kong 1968 strains of the influenza virus. Imagine my bitter disappointment when the *Journal of Experimental Medicine* rejected the article owing to a perceived 'lack of interest' to their readers. Granoff immediately suggested sending the article to George Hirst, now the editor of the journal *Virology*, who had discovered the haemagglutinin of influenza viruses. He would appreciate its significance. Indeed he did, and the paper was accepted with only minor changes for publication. The lesson for young scientists is not to be disappointed by initial rejection. You may just need to try a different, more appropriate journal. And then perhaps try again.

CHAPTER 7

VIROLOGISTS VISIT CHINA

Because both the Asian 1957 H2N2 and Hong Kong 1968 H3N2 influenza pandemics were first detected in southern China, this was surely the place to go to try to determine their source. That country's large populations of ducks, chickens, pigs and people certainly fitted with our growing hypothesis of likely factors. In mid-1972 Graeme Laver and I had the privilege of joining a group of Australian scientists visiting China to sample animals for influenza. We were probably the first Western influenza virologists to visit China after the start of the Cultural Revolution, and the experience was extremely scientifically rewarding.

The Asian H2N2 pandemic was first detected in humans in Kweiyang (Guiyang), Kweichow Province, in southern China in February 1957.[51] This virus differed from the descendants of the H1N1 Spanish influenza that was circulating in humans in 1956 in both its haemagglutinin and neuraminidase spikes. Humans worldwide had little or no immunity to this new H2N2 virus, and it spread rapidly overland through the Soviet Union and Hong Kong, and then by ship to the rest of the world, taking about six months to affect humans globally. A second wave struck many countries in the spring of 1958 and, altogether, 40–50 per cent of humans worldwide were affected, with an estimated death toll of 1.5 million people (see Figure 2.1).

Descendants of the Asian H2N2 influenza virus circulated globally from 1957 until 1968, when another new pandemic – the H3N2 Hong Kong strain – spread from China to Hong Kong, where it was first reported.[52] As its name tells, this H3N2 virus had a different haemagglutinin spike from the preceding H2N2 viruses but shared a related neuraminidase protein. Because some people were immune to the neuraminidase component, the Hong Kong pandemic spread comparatively slowly. In European countries it did not peak until December 1969. Nonetheless, the H3N2 virus resulted in an estimated global mortality of 1 million people. This showed that a change in the haemagglutinin spike was sufficient for a virus to cause a pandemic and that immunity to the N spike, while modulating the disease's severity, was insufficient to prevent its global spread.

Our dream at that time was to obtain permission to visit China to sample the hypothetical animal reservoir and to see if there was anything unique in the Chinese lifestyle or animal life pattern that would facilitate mixing (hybridisation) between human and animal influenza viruses. Laver and I also wanted to establish contact with Chinese virologists to share ideas and reagents (the antisera).

In early 1972 a group from what is today the Australian Institute of Medical Scientists (physicians, surgeons, dentists and public health officials) was working with the Chinese Medical Association to establish an exchange of scientific information in the different disciplines, and a group of them were about to visit China. Laver contacted the leaders of the Australian group and asked if the two of us could join them, explaining in some detail the importance of understanding the origin of pandemic influenza viruses. We also approached the WHO, which was delighted to support the visit. We were very excited when our invitations arrived. The Chinese Medical Association gave us permission to bring swabs and vials to sample animals and to bring serum for identifying the individual components on the surface of influenza viruses we might collect.

Although the 17 medical personnel from Australia were visiting at the invitation of the Chinese Medical Association, this was not considered an official delegation. Our trip was arranged by the China International Travel Service. We were there from 9 September to 4 October 1972, and our visit began in Hong Kong, where we visited Dr Wai-Kwan Chang, who had first reported the H3N2 pandemic there in 1968. We travelled by train to Canton (Guangzhou), then to Shihkiachwang (Shijiazhuang), Beijing, and then Tientsin (Tianjin). From then on, our travel was by air, taking us to Shenyang, Darien (Dalian), and Shanghai, except for the final leg to Hangchow (Hangzhou), which again was by train (Figure 7.1). The group had two guides and translators who took us to every meeting and to visit cultural sites in every city.

In 1972, shortly after the start of the Cultural Revolution, Chairman Mao Zedong's influence was very strong. At our first official meeting with the Chinese Medical Association in Guangzhou we were each given a copy of the *Little Red Book* of quotations from Chairman Mao and given a one-hour talk on the structure and merits of the new society. This was followed by presentations by Chinese medical authorities, emphasising their public health advances, including the eradication of sexually transmitted diseases and their current work on hepatitis and tuberculosis control. The merits of acupuncture for the control of pain and treatment of many disorders were explained, along with the wisdom of the mooted one-child family plan.

Our first impression of China was that it was definitely in its grey period: everyone wore a Mao jacket, pants and a hat of a grey-blue colour. We noticed too that personal transport was by bicycle. Throughout the tour we were met with enthusiastic friendliness not only by the officials guiding us but also by the staff of the many hospitals we visited, the virologists and the people in the street. In fact, on seeing us, people in the street would stop and clap, because they

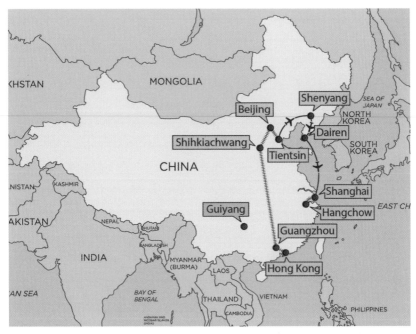

Figure 7.1 The cities we visited in China in 1972 are shown in orange. Our travel was mainly by train, although by air in the north. The city of Guiyang was where the Asian 1957 H2N2 pandemic was first detected.

had not seen Westerners since the start of the Cultural Revolution (Figure 7.2). We all wore big badges with our names in Chinese characters followed by 'Not Russian', an important distinction at a time when China was embroiled in a border dispute with the Soviet Union.

Laver and I were expected to accompany the rest of the group and visit hospitals in most of the cities we visited to observe the benefits of Chinese medicine and learn how it differed from Western medicine. We also had the opportunity to visit Chinese medicine stores and obtain herbal mixes for the treatment of influenza. As virologists, neither of us had ever been in an operating theatre to observe surgery. Yet on the second day of our visit to Canton we donned gowns and masks and witnessed major surgery with only acupuncture for anaesthesia. A woman was undergoing lung surgery, with her chest

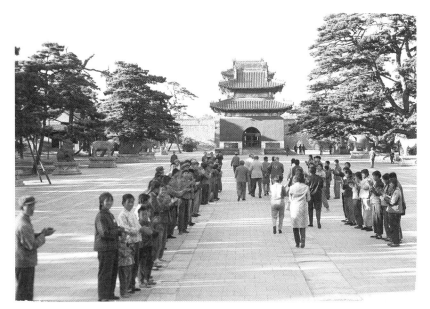

Figure 7.2 Wherever we went in China in 1972 people in the street stopped and clapped. Here we were visiting the North Tomb of Shenyang.

open and her heart visible. The woman actually spoke while the surgeon was working on her! It was truly amazing, and we could not quite believe that the woman was pain free. During the rest of the trip we observed acupuncture being used for pain control during surgery at each stop except in Shijiazhuang and Beijing, when Laver and I separated from the main group and met with virologists. We also saw it being used to treat a significant number of people with partly paralysed legs from poliomyelitis as well as those with arthritic conditions.

After witnessing the apparently extraordinary effects of acupuncture to control pain, I was keen to try it. So on one of our hospital visits, where people were being treated for polio-based paralysis, one of the physicians agreed to perform it on me. He explained through the interpreter that the acupuncture point for the

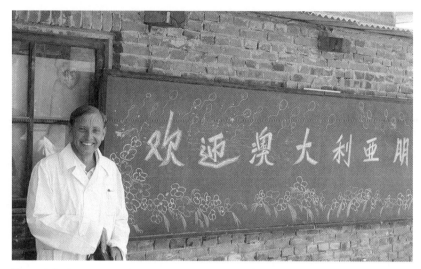

Figure 7.3 Graeme Laver beside the welcoming board at Shihkiachwang, which reads 'Welcome to Australian visitors'.

lower right side of the jaw, used during dental work, is between the thumb and index finger of the right hand. An acupuncture needle was duly inserted into my right hand and gently vibrated by hand. After a minute or so the physician inserted a needle into my lower jaw. I felt no pain. Was it a case of mind over matter? I will never forget Laver's question just as the acupuncture needle was put into my hand: 'What is the incubation period for hepatitis?' – a classic Laver comment. I was completely fine, but perhaps I should have asked about needle sterility beforehand.

Shijiazhuang had a huge military camp with its own pig farm, and an International Peace Hospital named after Norman Bethune, a physician from Canada. On the first evening of our stop there, we were feted at a traditional Chinese banquet with 13 different dishes, many speeches and many toasts of *gan bei* ('bottoms up') as we raised our glasses of *moutai* (a very strong, rice-based alcoholic drink). Needless to say, we were all quite tipsy through much of the evening (Figure 7.3).

One of the physicians from Melbourne received a lesson in cultural differences he would never forget. In Western society, children are taught that it is polite to eat all the food on one's plate. However, in China, a visitor's empty plate is always refilled by a Chinese host seated beside you. This young man kept emptying his plate, and his host kept refilling it, until his stomach could hold no more – with the inevitable result. The mess was cleared away as if by magic, but the young physician was so embarrassed that for the rest of the trip he ate only peanuts and fruit.

In our speeches we explained our hypothesis of the role of pigs in the origin of influenza pandemics. Our hosts said that they had many pigs and that in the morning we could sample them all. The next morning, after the requisite Mao lecture, a rather hungover group of Chinese, together with Laver and me, donned white coats and went to the piggery. In the first pen, a very healthy young adult pig was caught, and I used Dacron swabs to sample both nostrils, then collected blood from the animal's ear vein. The pig was released. Everyone stood back, so I asked for the next pig to sample. The interpreter very patiently explained to me that all pigs are the same. I equally patiently explained why we needed to test a number of animals. But it was not to be. Despite our repeated requests to collect samples from pigs and poultry, that one animal represented the total amount of animal sampling done on the entire visit. This was our first indication that the veterinary side of influenza research might not be as straightforward and cooperative as the human side.

Our disappointment about sampling animals was compensated for by the extremely warm welcome we received from Chinese influenza virologists in Beijing. We were most impressed when we arrived by train in Beijing at 4am and were met by Chu Chi Ming, head of virology at the institute, and his staff. Laver and I spent a whole day visiting the National Vaccine and Serum Institute (of the

Department of Biological Products), where we had each been invited to give a lecture, to be followed by extensive discussion. Chu had been trained in Cambridge and London, and he and his staff were very well informed about influenza.

We were somewhat concerned by then that our hypothesis that human pandemics of influenza originated from ducks and pigs might have been considered a slight to our Chinese hosts. Fortunately, however, there was open discussion and no hostility. Chu told us that the 1957 Asian H2N2 virus had first been isolated from outbreaks of influenza in humans in 20 counties in West Guizhou Province in February and March 1957. The general consensus among the 40 or so virologists at the meeting was that the virus was not from an animal source but instead arose by mutation from the late H1N1 strains. Chu described a group of 'bridging' strains that he had characterised, which he believed shared reactivity with both the late H1N1 and the early H2N2 viruses. We were delighted when Chu gave us samples of two viruses (A1/Loyang/3/57 and A1/Loyang/4/57) as well as a recent influenza B virus (B/Hunan/2/71). We gave Chu and his staff the antisera specific to the H and N of human, swine and equine influenza viruses.

The bridging strains of influenza viruses were subsequently shared widely with the influenza research community through the WHO. Once we returned to the laboratory in Memphis, we found that the A/Loyang viruses were sensitive to the inhibitors present in all sera. After we removed all the inhibitors, we found that they were in fact H1N1 influenza viruses. This meant that 'bridging strains' did not explain the origin of the H2N2 pandemic and that our animal reservoir hypothesis was still potentially valid.

Regarding the Hong Kong H3N2 virus, Chu said that the first virus was not isolated in mainland China until August 1968 but had been isolated in Hong Kong the previous month. This account differed from what we had been told in Hong Kong, illustrating a definite political sensitivity on such things. There, Chang had informed us that the H3N2 virus had first been isolated in mainland China. In discussions with virologists in many centres, including with a different Chang at Shenyang Medical College (where we had also shared reference reagents), it became apparent to us that although the Chinese believed influenza was important, it was not of major medical concern in China. There was no national influenza centre in China at that time, but 10 million doses of live, adapted Hong Kong/68 H3N2 vaccine had been produced by the National Vaccine and Serum Institute in Beijing for use in humans. The Chinese virologists gave no credence to our belief concerning the role of animals like ducks and pigs in the origin of pandemic influenza viruses of humans.

In Shenyang in the far north of China, our departure by air was delayed for a couple of days by rain and fog. But there was more than just water in the air. Since the weather was turning cooler, increased numbers of coal briquettes were being used for heating, and significant air pollution was becoming evident. As a farm boy, I also noticed some large duck farms and several live poultry markets in the southern cities. The importance of these observations, along with the memory of a banquet at a traditional roast-duck restaurant in Beijing, came together in some conclusions discussed in the next chapter.

In later years Graeme Laver often referred to this 1972 visit to China as 'the one-pig study'. The serum from the one pig from which we obtained samples did have antibodies to the H1N1 influenza virus, showing that it had been infected in the past with an influenza virus. However, the extracts made from herbs sold to treat influenza infection failed to inhibit the virus in our laboratory studies. Of course, they may well have analgesic effects.

We were greatly impressed by the willingness of the Chinese scientists to give us samples of their influenza viruses and openly discuss their information. Whether our visit played any part in the release of information about the re-emergence of the H1N1 virus A/USSR/90/77 (H1N1) in northern China in 1977, or the eventual acceptance of the hypothesis of an animal origin of pandemic influenza, we cannot ascertain. But there were many more exchange visits of scholars from China to our laboratories, and in November 1982 a meeting in Beijing – on the origin of pandemic influenza viruses – was sponsored by the Institute of Virology of the Chinese Academy of Medical Sciences and the Australian National University. These connections have continued to the present.

CHAPTER 8

HONG KONG HOTBED: LIVE BIRD MARKETS AND PIG PROCESSING

The first time I walked into a live bird market (LBM) in Hong Kong with my colleague Ken Shortridge from the University of Hong Kong in 1975, I realised that this was the place to study influenza. We did not have to go to the countryside in mainland China; here the farm animals came to us. The LBMs we saw in Hong Kong varied in size from a few cages of beautifully coloured yellow-brown chickens, known locally as 'yellow-haired chickens', tucked into an alley or under an overpass, to large city markets the size of huge supermarkets, with

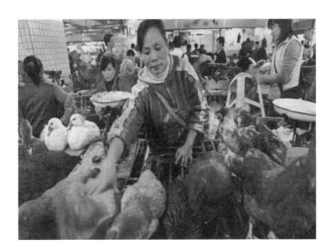

Figure 8.1 A classic live bird market in Central Market, Hong Kong, in the early 1970s, showing the mixture of different species in the same stall.

dozens of individual stalls selling live poultry. On the ground floor of these multi-storey city markets were stalls selling live or fresh fish, freshly slaughtered livestock (mainly pigs) and a vast variety of fresh vegetables; on the floors above, vendors offered household goods, clothing and furnishings for sale.

The tradition of LBMs goes back to the Ming Dynasty in the sixteenth century.[53] They developed in the hot climate of southern China as a means of making fresh meat available in an era before refrigeration, showing a keen popular understanding of the health risks of contaminated meat. The traditional LBMs in Hong Kong and southern China that were operating until 1997 are of most relevance to the influenza story. After the 1997 emergence of H5N1 bird flu, LBMs in Hong Kong changed dramatically (see Chapter 10), with a reduction in the number of markets and market size and a separation of species. In mainland China, however, LBMs have remained largely unchanged.

A large LBM in the city contained a wide variety of both land-based and aquatic birds (Figure 8.1). The land-based birds were mainly varieties of chicken (the yellow, the white and the silky chicken), with some quail and pigeons, and the occasional pheasant, chukar and guinea fowl. The aquatic birds included ducks of various varieties (white Peking ducks, khaki Campbell ducks, Muscovy ducks and a few wild ducks, mainly mallards) and a wide range of white, grey and black geese.

Just about every aspect of those LBMs promoted the spread of influenza viruses within and between species, as well as providing conditions for the development of new virus strains. I was sure I could see viruses rampantly mixing and hybridising before my very eyes. In some market stalls different species were kept in separate cages, but in others they shared cages. It was not uncommon to find ducks and chickens in the same cage. Cages were always stacked on top of each other, five or six high. While each cage had a water trough and litter pan, there was always spillage when the cages were opened, providing a wonderful opportunity for viruses to spread from cage to cage. Furthermore, while the market areas were regularly hosed down with water and were kept quite clean, individual stall owners rarely if ever emptied or cleaned their cages.

In Hong Kong, LBM stall owners obtained their birds from two central wholesale markets that in turn obtained their land-based birds by truck from farms in southern China or from the New Territories of Hong Kong. Aquatic birds mainly came by boat from the coastal duck farmers in China. Thus many of the birds I had seen being raised on farms in China would have ended up at LBMs in China or Hong Kong.

Once a chicken or quail arrived at a city's LBM, it was usually sold in one or two days. Ducks and geese took a little longer to sell (two to five days), and exotic species like the guinea fowl or pheasant might stay in the market for up to a week. Cages were constantly being topped up with newly arrived birds. Any one cage could hold any number of species, and some birds in each cage might be there for several days.

Customers shopping for fresh chicken or other poultry would survey the birds and sometimes handle them to feel their size and plumpness. The stall owner would then process the chosen birds on the spot, killing, defeathering and eviscerating them in the back of the stall. While the splattering of blood, feathers and entrails was kept to a minimum, it was inevitable that it would generate some aerosols – airborne particles of fluids or solids. Aerosols are effective carriers of viruses.

While the large city markets, and their LBMs, were convenient for the public, the combined effect of mixing species in a cage, stacking the cages, dirty cages, topping up bird numbers and processing birds on site created perfect conditions for virus transmission between birds and from birds to human customers, and for the development of novel influenza viruses.

I was reminded of the experiments we had done at Plum Island (Chapter 6), where two different influenza viruses were put into a turkey or a pig, and novel influenza viruses emerged. Biochemically, the effect of LBMs is akin to that of the polymerase chain reaction (PCR) technique used in scientific laboratories to replicate thousands of copies of genetic material or a virus.

***

In Hong Kong, the other animal of particular interest from an influenza perspective was (and still is) the pig. The 1918 Spanish influenza in the Americas spread into pigs and caused classical swine influenza year after year in the winter months. Had the H1N1 influenza virus in pigs spread globally? More specifically, was it present in pigs in southern China in the late 1970s? To answer these questions, Ken Shortridge and I set up a surveillance programme for influenza in pigs in Hong Kong.

The slaughtering of pigs was done at four slaughterhouses in Hong Kong, and the half-carcasses were delivered by truck, or even bicycle, to the meat stalls in the large central markets before daybreak. This meant there was much less contact between pigs and people than occurred in the LBMs. The pigs came from farms in Hunan, Jiangxi, Guizhou and Guangdong provinces in southern China, often crowded together in trucks or trains for up to three days. During this time, respiratory agents could spread, but the animals would not necessarily show disease signs before they arrived at the abattoir because the incubation time was not long enough. The humans at highest risk of infection were the stock handlers and butchers.

The length of time an influenza virus can survive in an animal carcass depends on the animal and the temperature of storage. If frozen, the virus can survive indefinitely; at refrigerated temperatures up to a week or more; and at room temperature for 1–2 days. Avian carcasses are more likely to have residual influenza viruses because these viruses are mainly present in the intestine and can contaminate the carcass during evisceration. In pigs the virus is mainly in the trachea and lungs, which are removed during evisceration. Cooking of poultry or pork destroys influenza virus.

After the emergence of the Hong Kong H3N2 influenza pandemic in 1968, the National Institutes of Health in the United States issued a request for the scientific community 'to elucidate the origin and possible control strategies for pandemic influenza'. Our group at St Jude Children's Research Hospital proposed collaborative studies on influenza in wild birds, poultry and pigs in both the United States and Hong Kong with Ken Shortridge, and we obtained funding for five years. These funds supported the long-term surveillance of wild migratory waterfowl in North America described in Chapters 4 and 5 and eventually led to the establishment of the ecological principles of influenza viruses described therein, which are now widely accepted. Most importantly, however, these funds supported the collaborations with Shortridge.

Shortridge had established a laboratory for influenza surveillance and research at the University of Hong Kong, and by 1977 we had found a plethora of influenza viruses belonging to different subtypes in LBMs, as well as a wide range of paramyxoviruses, including Newcastle disease virus (NDV), which can cause lethal disease in chickens. All of the virus isolates came from apparently healthy birds – mainly ducks, but some chickens and geese also.[54] We detected viruses in up to 10 per cent of the birds: half were influenza, and the rest were NDV. Thirteen different subtypes of influenza viruses were isolated, some related to the Hong Kong H3N2 of 1968 but most to influenza viruses from avian sources. Some, in fact, were closely related to influenza viruses from wild ducks in Canada, suggesting a global spread. Most of the influenza viruses we found were from cloacal rather than respiratory tract samples. Shortridge also found two different influenza viruses from the same duck, possessing the same haemagglutinin spike but different neuraminidase spikes. This suggested that influenza viruses were mixing their genetic material in the real world, as we had predicted from our research at Plum Island.

Studies in pigs at a slaughterhouse in Hong Kong in 1976 were equally rewarding. From 356 nasal swabs from apparently healthy pigs, we isolated 11 influenza viruses. All of the influenza viruses were H3N2, six being antigenically identical to the H3N2 1968 pandemic virus and five being similar to the H3N2 Hong Kong variant (A/Victoria/3/75) that was circulating in humans that year. So by 1976 the pandemic H3N2 influenza had disappeared from humans yet was still circulating in pigs.[55] The study also showed that the currently circulating influenza virus in humans had spread to pigs. The studies in pigs did not detect any of the avian influenza viruses found in LBMs in Hong Kong.

To be sure that the remarkably high diversity of influenza viruses found in birds in LBMs in Hong Kong was not a fluke, Shortridge continued the study for a second year. He not only confirmed the findings but also detected almost all known subtypes of influenza viruses, including those related to influenza viruses found in humans, horses and swine. Out of a total of the 136 influenza viruses isolated, 126 were from domestic ducks originally from China.[56] Thus, counterparts of influenza viruses found in wild ducks in the Americas were found in domestic ducks in China, suggesting that ducks constituted a global reservoir of influenza, and further supporting the idea that LBMs were a hotbed for the mixing of influenza genomes and the development of new influenza viruses, as well as for possible transmission to humans.

CHAPTER 9

SEARCHING THE WORLD, 1975–95

After we had successfully isolated influenza viruses from apparently healthy wild and domestic aquatic birds, numerous studies on avian and aquatic birds in Australia, Japan, the Soviet Union, Europe and the United States confirmed that influenza viruses are global in their distribution. Although some virus subtypes were more common in gulls than in ducks, and influenza viruses from Eurasia could be distinguished from those in the Americas, it was clear that influenza viruses could be found in aquatic birds worldwide. From the mid-1970s to the mid-1990s there was growing acceptance – among influenza virologists, ecologists and veterinarians – that wild aquatic birds were the reservoir of most subtypes of influenza A viruses. However, there was no smoking gun when it came to the transmission of these viruses to humans.

As early as 1952 the WHO had recognised that influenza was a global human health problem and created a worldwide network of surveillance. The WHO human influenza network supported our studies on influenza in pigs and ducks, to further our understanding of the sources of influenza viruses in humans.

St Jude Children's Research Hospital in Memphis became a collaborating centre in the WHO network in 1 January 1975, studying the ecology of influenza viruses at the human–animal interface. St Jude is known primarily as a cost-free children's cancer research hospital. It was established in 1962 by the entertainer Danny Thomas, who promised that he would build a monument to Saint Jude, the patron saint of lost causes, if he succeeded in show business. He kept his promise and duly consulted with Cardinal Samuel Stritch about the choice of an appropriate monument. The cardinal persuaded Danny against a statue – 'Birds will only poop on it, and it will not help humanity!' Instead he suggested building a small hospital in Memphis, the cardinal's first parish. Thomas's dream hospital was established, with great insight by its founders, as a place where clinical research and fundraising are integrated with the single goal of curing childhood cancer, at no cost to patients' families.

I am often asked, 'What does influenza have to do with cancer in children?' At the very first review of my influenza research at St Jude the chairman of the review panel asked me the same thing. I replied, 'Sir, do you know what kills our children at St Jude?' He said, 'Cancer, mainly childhood leukaemia.' I replied, 'No, it is the common infectious diseases like influenza, measles, the common cold that are our greatest killers, because all the therapies designed to kill cancer cells also inhibit children's immune responses to infectious disease.' At that time we did not have even one drug to treat influenza in children. My goal has always been to understand influenza and make new and better vaccines and drugs.

Thankfully, the review panel agreed and enthusiastically supported our role in the WHO.

***

I had opportunity to expand my global search for the source of influenza pandemics when I was invited later in 1975 to participate in a joint Soviet–American research programme on influenza. Since vast numbers of waterfowl breed in Siberia, we were delighted to participate in scientist exchanges between laboratories and in fieldwork in Russia.

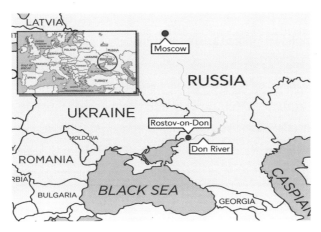

Figure 9.1 Influenza knows no boundaries. This map shows the two research sites where scientists from the former Soviet Union and from the US collaborated in 1975 to carry out influenza surveillance in wild aquatic birds on the Don River.

Early in the Northern Hemisphere spring, Bernard (Barney) Easterday from the University of Wisconsin, Madison, and I flew to Moscow and met our host, Dimitri L'vov, and his staff at the Ivanovsky Institute of Virology. We shared ideas and planned our upcoming fieldwork. The area for study was on the Don River, near Rostov-on-Don in southeastern Russia (Figure 9.1).

Migratory waterfowl overwintered in this region before returning to their breeding grounds in Siberia. Our method for obtaining waterfowl was to shoot them from high-powered aluminium boats. There were three people per boat: one to run the motor, one in the bow to shoot the birds, and one to pick up shot birds. We collected a wide range of herons, ducks, coots and other waterfowl. One afternoon I was out with two Russian colleagues, neither of whom spoke a word of English, and we were not having any success. It was bitterly cold. One of my colleagues waded towards shore and disappeared into the reeds. His long absence, at least 30 minutes, had me quite puzzled. Eventually he returned proudly displaying his find – a bottle of vodka that warmed us up very well.

Overall, 321 birds of 25 species were collected. In addition to taking swab samples from the throat and trachea, we collected tissue samples from the lungs, liver and intestines, and blood from the chest cavity. The same instruments were being used again and again to sample the different birds, so to minimise possible cross-contamination from one bird to the next, the instruments were dipped in 100 per cent alcohol, which was set alight. I was concerned about this method; I had been taught that this procedure needed to be repeated three times to ensure sterilisation. All became clear on the final afternoon, when we celebrated the success of the fieldwork. Once the vodka ran out, the leftover sterilising alcohol was brought out, and the party went on into the small hours.

The findings from the collaborative study confirmed that aquatic birds were indeed global reservoirs of influenza viruses. No influenza viruses were found in the 321 birds examined, but the sera of some of the birds had antibodies to many subtypes of virus.[57] Since influenza infection in birds lasts about the same time as it does in humans, finding actual virus particles in migratory birds requires being in the right place at the right time.

One question that was paramount at the time was how (and where) the many different subtypes of influenza A viruses are maintained in the 'off period', after the infection of a flock. One possibility was that they might be frozen in the polar regions. If so, perhaps the penguins in Antarctica were the ultimate influenza reservoir. To investigate this possibility, Frank Austin and Tony Robinson from the Health Research Council at the University of Otago, New Zealand, and I applied to the New Zealand Antarctic Programme to collect swab and blood samples from Adélie penguins (*Pygoscelis adeliae*), Antarctic skuas (*Catharacta antarctica*) and Weddell seals (*Leptonychotes weddellii*) to look for evidence of influenza infection. The project was approved for the Antarctic summer of January 1986, and the US Navy would fly us from

Christchurch to Scott Base (New Zealand's Antarctic research station) and back.

I will never forget being herded onto the Hercules aircraft by the loadmaster. Wearing all of our Antarctic clothing in case of an emergency, we waddled on board like penguins ourselves. Each seat was merely a webbing sling against the plane's outer skin. The centre of the plane was filled with huge crates, stacked from floor to ceiling. Even with earplugs the noise of the engines was tremendous. Several hours later I landed on an ice runway for my first time and disembarked to brilliant, clear skies. It was all very exciting.

Our first activity at Scott Base was survival training. On the second afternoon we were helicoptered out onto a snowfield on a glacier. Again we wore full Antarctic clothing and carried survival rations, sleeping bags and a folding snow shovel. Our instructions were to make an overnight shelter: we would be picked up the next day. Austin and I decided on an igloo rather than a snow cave and sheltered quite comfortably. The only issue was with my camera: I had not put it inside the sleeping bag, and the electronics froze up.

Samples were to be collected from the Adélie penguin and skua colonies at Cape Verde, on Ross Island. This was a considerable distance from Scott Base, so we were helicoptered there from Scott Base. The sight as the helicopter touched down was amazing. Adélie penguins appeared to fly out of the ocean between the coastal mounds of broken sea ice and strut in long lines to the vast nesting colony, where birds were busy disputing ownership of the available small stones.

We had understood that we were to stay in the one hut at the site, and were surprised to find out that folks from Radio New Zealand were occupying the hut for a couple of days. The radio team handed us tents for shelter. We worried we would not be warm enough, but those Antarctic tents were double walled, and with Antarctic sleeping bags as well, we had to open the entrance to keep cool.

Although Adélie penguins are only knee-high and seemed to wait for us to catch them, they are remarkably strong, and it was a struggle for one person to hold a bird still enough for the collection of swab samples from both ends and a blood sample. The skuas were caught with long poles at the edges of the penguin colony, where they hung around waiting to steal Adélie chicks for a meal, and were swabbed and bled before being released (Figure 9.2).

To collect samples from Weddell seals around Scott Base, we would scout for the seals on a snowmobile near the edge of the sea ice, then park the noisy machine some distance away and approach the seals on foot. Weddell seals are huge, often 3.5 metres long and weighing over 550 kilograms. The strategy was to creep up on a sleepy seal and pull a large hessian bag over its head. While one person held the bag in place, the other collected the blood sample from the seal's tail and then quickly took nose swabs as the bag was partially lifted. This sounds a bit risky, and we were quite apprehensive at first, but the seals turned out to be quite docile.

No influenza virus was isolated from over 200 samples from these three species, but approximately 10 per cent of the Adélies and skuas had antibodies in their sera, indicating that at some time they had been infected.[58] Antibodies to the H10 influenza subtype were detected in the Adélie penguins and to the N2 subtype in skuas. A paramyxovirus was also isolated from the Adélie penguins. No antibodies to influenza viruses were detected in Weddell seals.

The results from these studies were reminiscent of those from the earlier studies on migratory shorebirds on the Great Barrier Reef in Australia, revealing that both Adélie penguins and skuas are susceptible to influenza. More systematic sampling was necessary to isolate the viruses infecting these species, and in 2013 other research groups succeeded in isolating an H11N2 influenza virus from Adélie penguins and an H5N5 influenza virus from chinstrap penguins.[59]

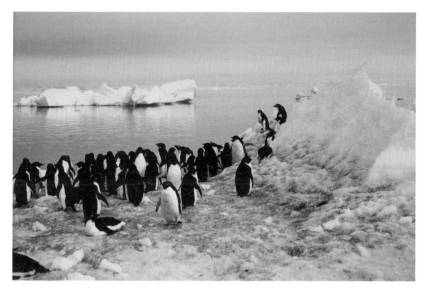

Figure 9.2 Adélie penguins at Cape Verde, Ross Island. Although these birds are only knee high it took two of us to hold them for sampling!

During this 20-odd year period (1975–96) influenza scientists and the WHO were actively pursuing collaborations with China on influenza surveillance in humans, pigs and poultry. Chinese scientists were equally interested in joining the global research community, for they realised that the WHO's global surveillance system for human influenza provided information that affected decisions about preparing influenza vaccines. China became an active participant in the WHO global programme in 1987, providing virus isolates from humans to compare with virus strains from other regions to determine if changes in vaccines should be recommended. By 1987 China was a major contributor. From 1987 to 2005, the strains recommended by the WHO for inclusion in vaccines worldwide contained at least one virus from China. Scientific exchanges were also fostered over this period, and in the early 1980s Chinese scientists, sponsored by the Chinese Ministry of Health, started to come on exchange visits to

PARAMYXOVIRUSES/ ORTHOMYXOVIRUSES

Paramyxoviruses are a different group of viruses from orthomyxoviruses (influenza viruses).

Their genetic structure is different – it is not segmented like influenza but does haemagglutinate red blood cells the way influenza does. Unlike orthomyxoviruses, the paramyxoviruses are genetically stable and do not show marked genetic variability.

These viruses cause respiratory disease, mumps and measles in humans, distemper in dogs, rinderpest in cattle and respiratory disease in poultry. The best known of the poultry diseases is Newcastle disease virus (NDV), which can vary in severity from mild to 100 per cent lethal. Like influenza viruses, the benign form of NDV and other paramyxoviruses occur in wild avian species.

WHO collaborating centres. These visits have continued to the present (Figure 9.3).

To further facilitate collaboration with the WHO, the Ministry of Health in China arranged visits for international scientists to its public health and municipal anti-epidemic stations in Beijing, Wuhan, Shanghai, Fuzhou and Shenzhen, in which I participated. The meetings were very productive, helping to establish strong collaborative ties and the sharing of ideas and methods for improving the surveillance and control of human influenza in China. Technical visits furthered understanding of the ecology of influenza in swine and poultry, including collaborations on surveillance of influenza in pigs in Kunming, Wuhan, Sichuan, Guizhou and Guangdong.

Under this programme, two scholars, Nannan Zhou and Lili Shu from Jangxi Medical College in Nanchang in southern China, worked

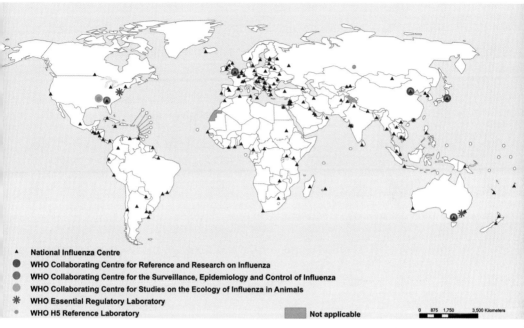

- ▲ **National Influenza Centre**
- ● **WHO Collaborating Centre for Reference and Research on Influenza**
- ◐ **WHO Collaborating Centre for the Surveillance, Epidemiology and Control of Influenza**
- ○ **WHO Collaborating Centre for Studies on the Ecology of Influenza in Animals**
- ✳ **WHO Essential Regulatory Laboratory**
- • **WHO H5 Reference Laboratory**
- **Not applicable**

0   875 1,750   3,500 Kilometers

Figure 9.3 The World Health Organization (WHO) Global Influenza Surveillance and Response System (GISRS) is made up of 144 national influenza centres that are the backbone of the network. There are six collaborating centres: four for reference and research; one for studies on the ecology of influenza in animals; one for the surveillance, epidemiology and control of influenza. There are four WHO essential regulatory laboratories, and 13 H5 reference laboratories. The collaborating centres meet twice yearly to make recommendations on the latest influenza virus to be included in vaccines. Courtesy of the World Health Organization

with their home university and provincial authorities to set up some experiments that Laver and I had hoped to carry out in 1970. The first study aimed to determine whether women who raised pigs in their homes had more evidence of influenza infections than women who did not.

Influenza viruses had been isolated weekly from the local women's hospital, and blood samples were taken from women who had come to the hospital with respiratory infections and did not raise pigs in their homes. The study showed that there was no difference in the frequency of human influenza infection between women who raised pigs in their homes and those who did not.[60] The study had three other important findings. Influenza outbreaks in the south central part of China were found to occur in two peaks: one in the winter months (November–March) and the other in the summer (July–September). The second outcome was that up to 25 per cent of the women raising pigs were found to have antibodies to H7, an avian influenza virus. The third outcome was a physical contribution to the WHO global network: one of the virus isolates from the women was found to be a representative of a novel H3N2 variant and was recommended by WHO for use as a vaccine strain for the entire world.

A second study was set up in 1996, involving 20 households that had one to three children per family and raised pigs and ducks in the same house. In these homes the pigs lived adjacent to the main living area, and the ducks had free range in the home. Influenza peaked in the households in winter, with a minor peak in the summer. Both humans and pigs exhibited a low incidence of the human Hong Kong H3N2 strain that was circulating in China at that time. Four different subtypes of influenza virus were isolated from the household ducks during the year of study. The overall incidence in the ducks was surprisingly low (0.9 per cent), much lower than we had found in the live bird markets.[61] One of the duck viruses was an H7N4, and again we found antibodies to these viruses in eight of 154 humans tested.

The main things we learned were that the incidence of influenza in household ducks was much lower than in ducks in the live bird markets (LBMs), and that although there was evidence that humans must have been infected with these duck viruses (because they had antibodies), the humans showed no disease signs. It appeared that influenza in the ducks was on rare occasions transmitted to children in the home but did not cause detectable influenza. Simultaneous surveillance of influenza viruses in the LBMs in Nanchang gave essentially the same findings as those from Hong Kong.

The studies in households in Nanchang contributed greatly to our understanding of the human–animal influenza interface. They not only yielded a human H3N2 influenza virus that was recommended by the WHO as a strain to include in human vaccines globally, but also confirmed that LBMs were much more likely sites of transmission to humans than households raising ducks and pigs.

CHAPTER 10

THE SMOKING GUN

While it was widely accepted by the 1990s that influenza in poultry and pigs could emerge from influenza viruses in wild aquatic birds, it was a stretch to persuade funding agencies that bird viruses could lead to influenza in humans. It had never happened, as far as anyone knew. But everything changed after the death of a child in Hong Kong in 1997.

On 21 May 1997 a three-year-old boy died in the intensive care section of Queen Elizabeth Hospital in Hong Kong from a severe influenza infection. The child had been perfectly healthy before the disease's sudden onset. Five days after admission he had a high fever and viral pneumonia. The pneumonia caused his lungs to fill with fluid, and he died.

Wilina Lim, head of the Public Health Laboratory for Hong Kong, isolated an influenza virus from samples collected from the boy's throat, but she could not identify it as one of the human influenza viruses in circulation; neither could the US Centers for Disease Control and Prevention (CDC) in Atlanta, Georgia. Lim sent the virus to Jan de Jong at the National Influenza Centre of the Netherlands, a longtime collaborator on influenza surveillance, for assistance with identification. De Jong and his colleague Ab Osterhaus knew that St Jude Children's Research Hospital had prepared antisera to the haemagglutinin and neuraminidase molecules of all the known influenza viruses. They contacted us and requested the antisera, which allowed them rapidly to identify the virus as similar to the avian H5N1 virus. This virus had, until then, been found only in chickens and ducks, and it killed up to 100 per cent of infected chickens. Thinking that perhaps the sample from the child had been contaminated somehow, de Jong visited the Hong Kong laboratory to ensure that the virus was not a laboratory contaminant. He and Osterhaus also examined the original swab – and confirmed that it contained the deadly H5N1 chicken influenza virus.

H5N1 infections were known to have broken out in three poultry farms in Hong Kong at this time, with a death rate among the birds of 70–100 per cent. However, the child who died was not known to have had any contact with these farms. Nowhere had H5N1 viruses been reported as infecting humans, so this first recorded case was a cause for enormous concern. Like my Dutch colleagues, I was concerned that this might be a pandemic warning.[62]

Fortunately, the H5N1 virus did not spread to the boy's family or to the staff taking care of him, and there were no immediate additional cases. But six months later, in November and December 1997, 17 more people became infected with H5N1 influenza, and five died. The WHO influenza network went onto high alert. A novel and very frightening influenza was emerging (Figure 10.1 and 10.2).

**

I heard about the outbreak on a Saturday morning. I was making compost in my garden when my wife, Marjorie, brought me the telephone. Nancy Cox, head of the Influenza Branch at the CDC, told me there were six more cases of severe influenza in Hong Kong, with half the victims in intensive care, and one person had already died. I was pretty certain this was the smoking gun we had been preparing for. I immediately called my colleague Ken Shortridge to ask if I could join him in Hong Kong and booked flights for the next day.

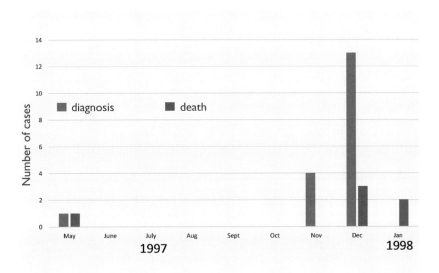

Figure 10.1 A timeline showing subsequent human cases of H5N1 influenza following the death of a child in Hong Kong in May 1997.

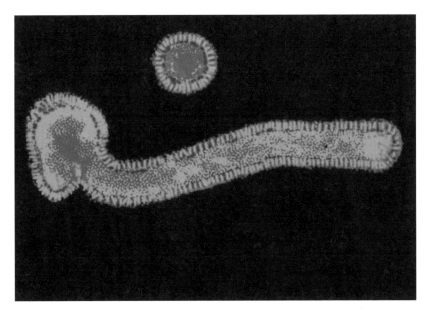

Figure 10.2 An electron micrograph of the H5N1 influenza virus from the three-year-old boy who died on 21 May 1997, showing the long thread-like (filamentous) and spherical morphology of the virus. Electron microscopy courtesy of Gopal Murti

On arrival in Hong Kong, I found everyone was preoccupied with the imminent transfer of the territory of Hong Kong from Britain back to China in July. Shortridge's laboratory at the University of Hong Kong was understaffed, for no new appointments were allowed during the transition period. It was obvious to me what we had to do: we had to sample the birds in the LBMs at once, and share the results with the staff in the agricultural and fisheries and the health departments. The sampling, the isolation of the viruses and injection into 10-day-old chicken eggs, and the testing of the eggs for the presence of viruses all take many skilled people, but skilled people were in short supply. So my first night in Hong Kong was spent on the telephone with young scientists from Japan and China whom I had trained, arranging for them to drop whatever they were doing and to join me as soon as possible, bringing all the gear we needed.

Two of the responsibilities that go with being a WHO collaborating centre on the ecology of influenza viruses are to train young scientists in research at the human–animal interface, and to collaborate with scientists internationally. One of my greatest collaborations occurred when Hiroshi Kida, a veterinarian from Hokkaido University in Japan, spent two year-long periods (1980–81 and 1986–87) as a visiting scientist in my laboratory. He is a strong proponent of the role of the pig in the genesis of human influenza pandemics, and of the theory that this occurs by reassortment between avian viruses and the previous human strains. He also strongly supports stamping out lethal influenza viruses in poultry rather than controlling them through vaccination. After returning to Hokkaido University he became chairman of his department and eventually director of the school. He is now a member of the Japanese Academy and head of the research centre for zoonoses at Hokkaido University. Perhaps his greatest gift to me was to send his brightest and best graduate students to St Jude to work in my laboratory. These were the trainees I called on to drop everything and come to Hong Kong in 1997.

The young virologists jumped to it. Toshi Ito and Ayato Takada in Japan immediately made arrangements to fly to Hong Kong. Yoshiro Kawaoka, one of the first post-doctoral fellows from Hokkaido and then a faculty member at St Jude, joined the group, as did another virologist, Peng Gao, a postdoctoral fellow from China. These four, along with Shortridge and myself, made up the initial team. We all realised the significance of what was happening in Hong Kong and all wanted to be part of the group working on this emerging influenza virus. One of the scientists was quite worried about coming through airports with a suitcase full of syringes and tubes of liquid and additional gear, but luckily his luggage was not examined.

Inviting a group of young scientists into an influenza hot zone caused me no small amount of worry. In preparation for any emergency, we had obtained the H5N1 influenza virus from the first human case (the boy in Hong Kong) and had prepared a concentrated vaccine, treated with formalin to kill all the viruses in it. The day the whole team arrived in Hong Kong, we decided to vaccinate ourselves by dripping the vaccine into our noses. I duly lay down on the examining table to let John Nicholls from Hong Kong drip the vaccine into my nose. As he was doing so he asked, 'Now, are you *sure* this H5N1 vaccine is dead?' I felt one of those moments of deep unease. Although we had tested the vaccine twice in developing chicken eggs, it had not been tested in an animal or human. I stood up and decided we would wait another day before vaccinating the rest of the team. I would serve as a guinea pig for one day.

As it turned out, none of the group got influenza, despite handling infected birds. Years later, when I participated in an H5N1 vaccine trial, I responded with a very high level of antibodies – a result of the fact that I had been vaccinated before. (An alternative way to avoid infection while working in the LBMs or the laboratory would have been to take a daily dose of the drug rimantadine, which inhibits viral replication. The group opted to use the vaccine instead.)

In 1997 there were more than a thousand LBMs in Hong Kong. With approval of the Department of Agricultural and Fisheries, Shortridge and the international team concentrated our studies on the six large municipal markets of Kowloon and the major districts of Hong Kong, including the markets that the patients' families had visited prior to developing influenza. These included Central Market and Smithfield on Hong Kong Island. At Central Market, the species present were typical – chickens, ducks, geese, quail and pigeons, with a few guinea fowl, chukar and pheasants – and all of the birds were healthy. None had ruffled feathers or was lying down. With the permission of the agricultural authorities and the stall owners we collected throat and faecal samples.

Two challenges arose during the investigations. One was the availability of the 10-day-old fertile chicken eggs known to be free of all known disease agents and called specific pathogen free (SPF) that we needed for isolating the influenza viruses. These were initially supplied by our colleagues at Agriculture and Fisheries, but our needs soon outstripped what they could supply. In the end, fertile eggs were flown in from Australia. The other challenge was the limitations of the laboratories in the Department of Microbiology at Queen Mary Hospital, Hong Kong University. These facilities were not designed to handle huge numbers of potentially deadly viruses. For one thing, there was only one biosafety cabinet (with filters and air flow to protect both the investigator and the laboratory from contamination by the virus under study). Departmental staff quickly recognised the need for a swift upgrade and organised a team of construction workers. They worked through the Christmas and (Western) New Year holidays modifying a laboratory with the required specialised air filters, and biosafety cabinets were flown in from the United States, installed and tested.

We had previously provided reference sera for identifying the haemagglutinin and neuraminidase components of all known influenza viruses. Two days after the first samples were injected into fertile eggs, the extensive preparations and careful methods started to bear fruit. We isolated several influenza viruses from the apparently healthy chickens (and some ducks) from the LBM at Hong Kong's Central Market. The very first virus was a surprise – it was H9N2, not H5N1. As the tests went on, H5N1 and H9N2 were found to be the major influenza viruses present. The significance of finding H5N1 was obvious, but we did not initially realise the relevance of H9N2.

We reported immediately to the health and the agricultural and fisheries departments that H5N1 was present in the LBMs. Their question, of course, was whether this was indeed the virus that was spreading to humans with severe and even fatal results. To answer this question, we now had the more precise tools of genetic sequencing at our disposal. We extracted the virus's genetic material, treated it so that it was denatured, and sent it on the next flight back to Memphis. In the lab there, over the weekend, we were able to read the genetic sequences of both the human and chicken H5N1 influenza viruses. Specifically, we determined the genetic code for their haemagglutinin proteins.

I flew back to Hong Kong on the Monday afternoon with the answer. The H5 components of the chicken and human virus samples were essentially identical. The virus from the birds in the LBM was the highly virulent H5 influenza virus.

In the meantime, Shortridge and the international team had sampled all six LBMs. The H5N1 influenza virus was present in all of them, with up to 20 per cent of chickens affected.[63] We knew we had identified the likely source for the human influenza outbreak.

The humans infected with H5N1 'bird flu' ranged in age from one year to 60. Early symptoms were typical of influenza, including high fever and upper respiratory tract infection, but in over half the sufferers the disease progressed and people developed severe pneumonia with vomiting, diarrhoea and liver and kidney dysfunction. Six of the 18 infected people died.

Margaret Chan, head of the Health Department in Hong Kong during this period, convened a panel consisting of senior staff of all the relevant government departments, including health, environmental services, and agriculture and fisheries. Also included were senior university scientific staff and representatives from WHO laboratories in Geneva, Atlanta and Memphis. This impressive lineup showed Chan's recognition of the importance of having all interested parties on board to draw together all available information and develop a plan.

After all the information was presented, it became obvious that a deadly H5N1 influenza virus of chickens was spreading to humans and causing up to 30 per cent mortality. The disease must be spreading through the LBMs, for the markets were where the public had contact with live poultry. The huge concern was that the virus might start to spread from human to human, which could lead to a global catastrophe. The tipping point was when a poultry farm in the New Territories of Hong Kong was found to have dead birds that were diagnosed with bird flu, and these birds were traced to the LBMs.

After many meetings, and before more people had become infected, Chan and the panel recommended to the health secretary that all LBMs be closed and all poultry in Hong Kong be culled and buried. This was a huge task and an enormous disruption to citizens' lives, but the health effects were dramatic. There were no more human cases of H5N1 bird flu, and that particular strain of H5N1 virus was stamped out.

The episode was not without its lighter moments. During the massive culling of poultry, I played decoy at one stage for the press. The cull began on 27 December in the wholesale market in Kowloon. The gates to that market were closed and the press of the world was outside them, clamouring for interviews and photographs. Inside, government staff were busy, along with Shortridge, Klaus Stohr from the WHO and the rest of our team collecting samples from a representative number of birds from each truck as they were euthanised. It was a prolonged, unpleasant business and when we finished the road outside the market was still packed full of media vehicles, with reporters, photographers and TV cameras everywhere.

We really didn't want them photographing great piles of dead chickens, which would have been very upsetting to most people, so it was decided that I should distract the press with a little speech about the public benefits of what we were doing and how we had to stop the killer H5N1 influenza virus before it started spreading among humans. A bright yellow Jeep was positioned as my platform. and the gates were opened. I spoke, and after a short question-and-answer session the Jeep drove off, with me on board, ostensibly to the next poultry-culling site. We were duly followed by an entourage of TV vans. After a very short ride, the yellow Jeep turned into a warehouse, where I switched to a small car and drove away. I had drawn the press from the team, which meanwhile made its way to the next site unhindered.

The next day I developed a high fever. I was alarmed that I might have picked up the virus, but fortunately my throat swab samples tested negative. Perhaps the vaccine I had indeed provided protection.

One of the puzzling aspects of the outbreak was the fact that there were no sick or dead chickens in the LBMs when humans were becoming infected, yet we isolated the virus from up to 20 per cent of the chickens we sampled. And the H5N1 virus that we isolated from those chickens was 100 per cent lethal when we put it back into chickens in our high-containment laboratory. We wondered whether stall owners might have been hiding dead birds or had whisked away all the sick birds before the markets opened in the morning. But no sick or dead birds were sighted.

The other possibility was that the chickens had been protected by the presence of another influenza virus circulating in the LBMs. We had earlier found an H9N2 influenza virus, along with H5N1, in the chickens sampled in each of Hong Kong's LBMs. While that virus causes little or no disease in chickens, it has contributed to the makeup of the deadly H5N1 influenza virus through the mixing of genetic material. Because it shares internal components with the H5N1 virus, the H9N2 virus was probably providing some cross-protection to the chickens.

Understandably, closure of the LBMs in Hong Kong, with Chinese New Year approaching, caused outrage among the stall owners. However, to their credit, and despite considerable public pressure, health authorities kept them shut for seven weeks until strategies could be devised to reduce the risk of H5N1 being reintroduced. To start with, all markets – wholesale and retail – were thoroughly cleaned and disinfected, and a regime of market inspections was introduced. Every retail market was ordered to empty completely for one day per month. Wild waterfowl were banned from the markets, and domestic waterfowl were to be brought into a separate wholesale market for processing, after which they would be sold as freshly killed birds in the retail markets. Wooden cages for the transport of poultry were replaced by plastic ones, and a giant cage-washing machine was installed to clean every cage before it was reused.

The strategy for cleaning the LBM and killing infectious agents such as influenza viruses involves cleaning to remove all organic matter (faeces), then washing with detergent and treatment with a chemical disinfectant. Detergents destroy influenza viruses, and chemical disinfectants kill any residual infectious agents.

The poultry farms supplying these markets were also inspected, as were the birds on each truck, and any dead or sick birds were tested on the spot for the presence of the influenza virus. Perhaps most importantly, the poultry traders and stall owners were compensated quite generously for each bird culled. This policy meant that these stakeholders became part of the solution in the control of H5N1 bird flu and did not try to hide diseased birds or shortcut the cleanup.

These strategies succeeded in keeping H5N1 out of the LBMs in Hong Kong from late 1997 until 1999, when the bird flu virus was detected once again, and the whole process of LBM closure, depopulation, cleaning and compensation was repeated.

We were hugely concerned, of course, that H5N1 would spread beyond China. We had discovered that novel influenza viruses could emerge in avian species and spread directly to humans without passing through an intermediate animal such as a pig. Fortunately, the H5N1 virus did not seem to have the ability to spread from human to human, but we feared that if we didn't prevent its spread to humans, the virus would eventually acquire this ability, and the resultant outbreak would be much worse than the Spanish influenza of 1918.

CHAPTER 11

BIRD FLU: THE RISE AND SPREAD OF H5N1

The key questions after the initial stamping out of the H5N1 influenza virus in Hong Kong in 1997 were, where had this chicken-killing virus come from? How had the virus gained the ability to spread to, and kill, humans? Would it reappear and spread? Had the H5N1 influenza become established in a reservoir animal population in which it was not so deadly? What was the role of H9N2? And finally, would H5N1 spread beyond China? The global influenza research community needed answers to these questions so that both agricultural and human health officials could be prepared should the virus 'take wing'.

The H5N1 influenza virus, which became known as bird flu, had appeared first in geese in Guangdong Province in China in the autumn of 1996. Outbreaks of severe disease were resulting in the deaths of up to 40 per cent of goose populations. Attempts to trace the virus's origins have largely failed, owing to the lack of material from before that time, because back then there was little or no interest in Asia in isolating influenza viruses from wild migratory birds. Based on what we know now, the H5N1 goose virus probably came from the wild ducks, in which it caused no disease. After the virus spread to domestic geese, it changed from a mild to a deadly strain by a process that we still do not fully understand. Then somehow the Guangdong

H5N1 influenza virus spread from geese to chicken farms, leading to lethal outbreaks in Hong Kong in March 1997, and then in farms in neighbouring areas in April and May.[64] In hindsight, it seems likely that chickens from infected farms had been sent to LBMs in Hong Kong.

Although there were sick geese in Guangdong Province in 1996, and sick and dead chickens in the adjacent territories of Hong Kong the following year, there were no reports of sick humans in either region at those times. The first human death was the child in Hong Kong in May 1997. Comparison of the H5N1 virus from Guangzhou geese with the virus isolated from the boy showed that the virus from the child had acquired new internal components. Even the neuraminidase (N1) spike was different. The only component that was consistent was the haemagglutinin (H5) spike. How had the child's virus acquired this other material?

As with other infectious diseases, crowding of different species together provides the perfect conditions for viruses to mix their genes, and this is probably what happened in Hong Kong's LBMs in the first half of 1997. The genes of the goose H5N1 virus mixed with those of other viruses. In this process the goose H5N1 virus probably acquired pieces of genetic code from the several other influenza viruses carried by the wide variety of birds, and those pieces enabled H5N1 to spread to humans. Virologists now believe that the key virus was H9N2, because it was also prevalent in the LBMs.[65] The H9N2 influenza virus was the ghost in the background (Figure 11.1).

Before the emergence of H9N2, which we nicknamed 'the enabler', no human had been infected with H5 viruses anywhere in the world, despite their causing deadly outbreaks in chickens in different parts of the world. Large outbreaks of lethal H5N2 influenza viruses had hit chicken farms in Lancaster County, Pennsylvania, in the 1980s. Millions of chickens were culled, and quarantine zones were established around the area. Throat swabs from the workers culling

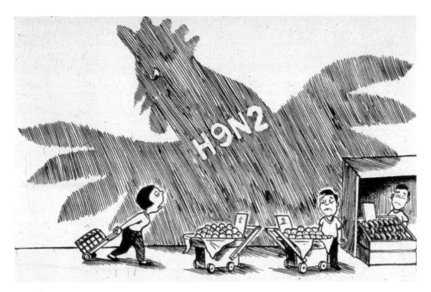

Figure 11.1 In April 1999 the *South China Morning Post* published a cartoon that accurately depicted H9N2 as the ghost in the background. Reprinted with permission from the *South China Morning Post*

the birds yielded the H5N2 influenza virus, but follow-up swabs taken the next morning came up clean. These findings showed that avian H5 viruses had been inhaled by the workers but could not multiply in the human body. It is noteworthy that the virus responsible for the second bird flu, in 2013, also contained numerous components of H9N2.

Meanwhile, back in Hong Kong in 1998, strict procedures were put in place to reduce the possibility of reacquiring the H5N1 virus from poultry farms in Hong Kong or China: registration of all farms providing birds to LBMs; frequent testing of birds; and the separation of geese and ducks in the wholesale markets. Thanks to these measures, no H5N1 influenza virus was detected in Hong Kong markets throughout 1998.

However, in 1999 the virus was found in samples taken from under goose cages in the waterfowl wholesale market. This H5N1 goose influenza virus was not the same as the original Guangdong goose

H5N1 virus, nor was it the H5N1 virus from humans. It had picked up internal components from other influenza viruses in southern China. The number of H5N1 isolates from the waterfowl market increased from four in 1999 to 18 in 2000 and was much higher again in 2001, indicating that the waterfowl were a major source of H5N1 influenza viruses. These findings led eventually to the closure of the waterfowl wholesale market in Hong Kong, and to all ducks and geese being sold in the processed and chilled state (imported from mainland China).

Despite the presence of H5N1 in the waterfowl wholesale markets, the chicken LBMs remained free of the virus until May 2001, when yet another H5N1 strain with novel internal components appeared, resulting in a repeat of the extreme measures of 1997: all markets were closed and cleaned and all birds culled. Additional steps were put in place to control further reintroductions. Quail were banned from the LBMs, as they were often infected with both H9N2 and H5N1 influenza viruses, and rest days were mandated, when all of the retail stalls were required to completely empty their cages of birds and sell killed and dressed poultry only (usually to restaurants). That allowed all the markets throughout the city to be closed for a day for thorough washing and disinfection.

It was apparent that H5N1 was present in the aquatic birds that visited or lived on the farms supplying Hong Kong with its waterfowl, and that domestic ducks had become the main source of the virus. It is not known exactly when the goose H5N1 influenza virus spread to ducks, but since the birds are raised in adjacent areas and transported together to Hong Kong's LBMs and later to its waterfowl wholesale market, it is not surprising. The problem with domestic ducks is that many varieties are asymptomatic when infected with the H5N1 virus – the very virus that kills 100 per cent of chickens that are infected. In fact, most varieties of duck are unaffected by the H5N1 virus infection, which makes them the Trojan horse of H5N1 influenza: apparently

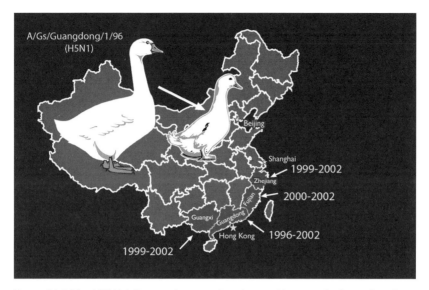

Figure 11.2 The H5N1 influenza virus was first detected in geese in Guangdong in 1996 and caused up to 40 per cent of deaths in these birds. Subsequently the virus spread to domestic ducks in many of China's coastal provinces, where it caused largely inapparent disease.

healthy ducks could bring the H5N1 influenza virus into the LBMs and spread it to other poultry and to humans. However, even in ducks, the H5N1 viruses showed enormous variability. Some of the more recent strains make ducks sick and affect their nervous system, causing them to swim in circles or turn their heads backwards.

And the virus wasn't just appearing among Hong Kong's local waterfowl suppliers. Farms in coastal Chinese towns in Guangdong, Guangxi, Fujian, Zhejiang and Shanghai provinces were sampled from 1999 to 2002, and their apparently healthy ducks were found to be infected with H5N1 viruses, showing that those viruses were widespread (Figure 11.2).[66] The study also clearly showed that the H5N1 viruses continued to evolve over time by obtaining components from other influenza viruses, as suspected, and they were now lethal to mice (tested experimentally). If they could kill mice (mammals), they could potentially infect humans.

In December 2002 there were outbreaks of H5N1 influenza in nature parks in Hong Kong, which killed exotic aquatic birds, including flamingos, as well as ducks and geese. Many parks were affected, indicating that the H5N1 had spread to wild, free-flying migratory birds. This particular virus strain was a lethal one for ducks (as experiments confirmed): infected ducks developed the characteristic head twisting and neurological signs of disease and had to be euthanised.

***

During the following Northern Hemisphere winter of 2003–04, the H5N1 influenza virus finally took wing and spread across Asia, almost simultaneously infecting birds in Vietnam, Thailand, Indonesia, South Korea, Japan, Cambodia and Laos. That virus had acquired several new internal components and was designated genotype Z (the mixture of gene segments in an influenza virus can vary with gene segments acquired during reassortment/hybridisation). It still contained the original haemagglutinin protein from geese in Guangzhou but had acquired all of its seven other components, also from aquatic birds in China.[67] This H5N1 virus had become entrenched in domestic ducks and then re-infected wild ducks, which contributed to its spread. These H5N1 Z genotype viruses also caused human infections in all of these countries. By 2004, 29 people were infected in Vietnam, and 20 people had died; in Thailand 17 people were infected and 12 people died.

H5N1 remained active in China and spread later in 2004 to Malaysia. All of the H5N1 influenza outbreaks in these different countries could be traced back to the Z genotype from China, but not to the same part of the country. For example, the poultry viruses that infected people in Thailand and Vietnam could be traced back genetically to the H5N1 virus from Hong Kong; the viruses infecting Indonesians could be traced to Yunnan Province in southern China.

So how did these H5N1 viruses that were actively evolving in ducks in China spread nearly concurrently across Asia? The easy explanation is that they were transmitted by wild migratory ducks and other waterfowl. In Hong Kong, the Z strain had been isolated from a dead little egret (*Egretta garzetta*), two dead grey herons (*Ardea cinerea*), a black-headed gull (*Chroicocephalus ridibundus*), a tree sparrow (*Passer montanus*) and a peregrine falcon (*Falco peregrinus*). However, domestic ducks are raised and fed in the open, and infected ducks shed the influenza virus into the water in their faeces as they swim. The dead wild birds could have been scavenging on a domestic duck farm. The other likely method of spread was through the trade in domestic birds across the region. It's likely both of these methods contributed to the spread of the Z strain of H5N1 influenza viruses across Asia. Restrictions on the movement of all live birds and poultry products were put into place in Hong Kong after 2004.

The really long-distance spread did not occur until after May 2005, when there was a major die-off of bar-headed geese (*Anser indicus*), gulls, cormorants and ruddy shelducks (*Tadorna ferruginea*) at Qinghai Lake in western China, from which the H5N1 influenza virus (Z strain) was isolated. The virus then spread to Mongolia, Siberia, Turkey, the rest of Europe and Africa. There are unconfirmed reports of commercial farming of bar-headed geese in the vicinity of Qinghai Lake, but there is little doubt that migratory birds were the main agents in the long-distance movement of the H5N1 viruses. In each country affected, swans, geese and other wild waterfowl died, and the virus spread to commercial poultry and to humans. For example, in 2006 there were eight people infected in Azerbaijan, with five deaths; in Turkey 12 people were infected, and four died.

There are two major strategies for controlling an emerging infectious disease agent that is a threat to human and animal health. The first is to stamp it out by a combination of culling (of animals!), quarantine, cleaning and disinfection, and compensation. Destroyed animals are incinerated, composted or buried. This policy is continued until there is no detectable virus in the region. The second strategy is to cull infected flocks and then administer influenza vaccine to the agent of spread (other birds), to prevent further spread and to control disease signs.

When a disease agent is first detected and confined to a small area, the first option is usually adopted. All the countries in Europe that were alerted to the spread of H5N1 bird flu looked to stamp it out, as did Japan and South Korea. All were successful at stamping out the initial H5N1 virus, as well as the later varieties that were reintroduced.

In countries where the flu was widespread before control measures could be adopted, combined culling and vaccination measures were adopted. China (including Hong Kong), Vietnam, Indonesia and later Egypt adopted this strategy, using the highly effective poultry vaccines that were rapidly developed. These vaccines have drastically reduced the incidence of H5N1 influenza in people and poultry. In Hong Kong, where all imported poultry for LBMs must now be vaccinated and tested for immunity to H5N1, no bird flu has been detected for many years.

The effectiveness of the H5N1 bird flu vaccine programme for poultry was dramatically illustrated in Vietnam. In 2005 there were 61 human cases of H5N1 influenza and 19 deaths, and the virus was prevalent in the LBMs there. After near-universal vaccination of poultry, including all domestic ducks, the number of human cases fell to zero in 2006, and no H5N1 was detected in LBMs. The number of people infected with the H5N1 virus in China also plummeted after widespread use of the poultry vaccine.

The bad news is that in those countries that opted to use the vaccine, the virus has become endemic. This means that H5N1 influenza viruses are persistently present in China, Vietnam, Indonesia and Egypt. How this happened is again clearly illustrated in Vietnam. The difficulty is in keeping all poultry fully vaccinated. By 2007 there were eight cases of H5N1 influenza in humans, with five deaths; in 2008 there were six cases and five deaths. Because the H5N1 virus can sicken and kill chickens, farmers are willing to vaccinate each new batch of chickens. However, duck farmers can be reluctant to shoulder the burden of vaccinating their birds, because the virus causes no disease in ducks. Duck farmers might well ask, 'Why should I spend money on a vaccine against a virus that causes no disease in my ducks?' And yet of course ducks are silent carriers of the virus.

Furthermore, although vaccination is effective at reducing human and poultry disease, in the long term it encourages the development of virus strains that the vaccine can't control. The bottom line is that while short-term vaccination to control virus spread can be useful in conjunction with culling, the long-term use of vaccination leads to virus persistence.

In order to minimise the spread of diseases that are a threat to animal health and thereby to the world food supply, nations belonging to the World Organization of Animal Health are obliged to notify that body when a reportable disease occurs. H5N1 bird flu is of course one such reportable disease. But one of the consequences of reporting the disease is that a country effectively invites all other countries to place an embargo on related products from that country. For the H5N1 virus, the embargo may include all live or processed poultry products, including frozen carcasses, and even feathers and duck down. Millions of dollars of income may be at stake. As a result, there is a tendency to hold back the information, and thus humans in Asia were serving as indicators of poultry disease – the proverbial canaries in the coal mine. Although the H5N1 influenza virus was isolated from geese in Guangdong in 1996, it wasn't until the first person contracted H5N1 bird flu, when staff from the CDC began searching for a possible source, that knowledge of the virus in geese was revealed.[68]

Another example of a reluctance to share information concerned our research to determine how quickly H5N1, present in geese and ducks in the coastal areas of China, would appear in the LBMs of central China and become a potential threat to humans in that region. Jiangxi Medical University in Nanchang and our team from St Jude Children's Research Hospital had a long-term surveillance programme for influenza under way in the LBMs of central China in order to answer this question. From the monthly sampling of poultry in a Nanchang LBM we isolated a wide spectrum of influenza viruses, including H9N2 influenza virus with four different internal compositions. Then, in February 2000, an H5N1 influenza virus was isolated from one quail and four chickens. The birds looked perfectly healthy, and there were no dead birds in the market. The H5N1 influenza virus was next isolated at the Nanchang LBM from three quail in May, suggesting that the farms supplying the markets were not widely infected (Figure 11.3).

Comparison showed that the Nanchang H5N1 virus was essentially identical with the H5N1 viruses from Hong Kong, meaning that these deadly H5N1 viruses were now in Nanchang's LBMs. We immediately sent a written report back to the Jiangxi Medical University and asked our colleagues to inform the agricultural authorities in the province and in Beijing. The university was most interested and sent the information forward as requested, but soon afterwards the entire surveillance programme was shut down. Stopping the influenza surveillance at Jiangxi Medical College was understandable because the laboratory did not have the high-containment facilities to protect the personnel from a deadly virus. What was surprising was that nothing was done to close the LBM or to reduce the spread of the virus. In fact information on H5N1 influenza in the regions of China was not reported to the World Organization for Animal Health until 2004.

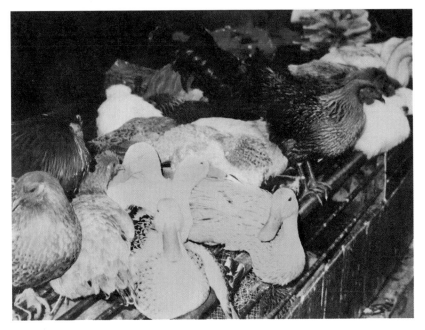

Figure 11.3 A typical live bird market in Nanchang, Jiangxi province, south-central China, showing the ready mixing of bird species. This was where the H5N1 influenza virus was first detected in February 2000.

That year, I was one of the authors of a scientific article reporting that a man and his family from Hong Kong had contracted influenza after visiting relations in Fujian Province in China.[69] The eight-year-old daughter died of pneumonia while in Fujian; the 33-year-old man also became ill in Fujian and died of viral pneumonia after returning to Hong Kong, and a nine-year-old boy suffered severe influenza but eventually recovered. The influenza viruses isolated from the family belonged to the Z strain – the one found in wild birds that had begun killing ducks in nature parks in Hong Kong two years earlier. The absence of virus in the Hong Kong LBMs when the family became infected strongly suggests that they were infected in Fujian.

The article arose from a collaborative study between staff at St Jude and the University of Hong Kong. The deaths of two members of the same family, and the properties of these viruses in mice experimentally infected with them, indicated to us that the viruses could be a threat to humans (as well as to poultry), so we published the information to alert Chinese health officials of the need to prepare vaccines and implement strategies to reduce the spread. There was no vaccine available for the Z type of H5N1.

Almost as soon as the information was published, Chinese authorities tried – but failed – to have the article removed from the journal. The Ministry of Health and the Ministry of Agriculture in China, in conjunction with the World Health Organization (WHO), called a meeting of China's leading scientists and the influenza experts in the WHO's influenza network to discuss the virological and epidemiological situation in China regarding H5N1. They met in Beijing on 4–8 December 2006.

The Ministry of Health was greatly concerned about the Z strain spreading from infected humans to others in China, while the Ministry of Agriculture was focused on conveying its view that H5N1 influenza viruses were not as widespread in China as the journal article made out. The really important underlying question for the whole meeting was raised by Nancy Cox from the CDC in Atlanta, who asked the presenter from the Ministry of Agriculture, 'If there is little or no influenza in poultry in China, how do you explain the 20 human cases that were reported recently from your country? Do we have human-to-human transmission of the current Z strain of H5N1?' The officials did not dispute the 20 recent human infections but adamantly denied human-to-human transmission. They believed that they had created H5N1-free zones by using the poultry vaccine.

The use of the frequently updated poultry vaccine in China has been successful in keeping the number of human infections low, with zero infections in 2017. However, the H5 viruses have continued to evolve, with H5N6 causing both human and poultry infections. The domestic duck continues to be the underlying problem. H5N1 viruses are endemic in domestic ducks, with occasional spillover into domestic chickens and humans. There is currently no incentive or realistic strategy to eradicate the H5N1 influenza virus. It will take many human deaths, or human-to-human transmission of an evolving H5N1 (or other lethal influenza virus), to bring about the closure of LBMs and to force the authorities to take stronger steps to eliminate lethal influenza viruses from domestic waterfowl in the region.

CHAPTER 12

THE FIRST PANDEMIC OF THE 21st CENTURY

With the continuing spread of H5N1 influenza virus and its ability to keep changing by picking up pieces of other influenza viruses from the wild bird reservoir, the world's influenza experts – including myself – were convinced that the next influenza pandemic in humans would be caused by an H5N1 virus. Our thinking was that it was only a matter of time before the H5N1 virus acquired the ability to spread not only from poultry to people but also from person to person. Since up to 60 per cent of people infected with H5N1 died, this scenario was exceedingly alarming. We all decided that we needed vaccines and medicines prepared and ready for immediate use if a virus 'hotspot' flared up, and we considered the various biomedical and public health strategies for preventing and treating influenza outbreaks.

The ability to modify influenza viruses in the laboratory was a major breakthrough, allowing the quick preparation of safe vaccines. This process entails making a H5N1 virus safe for vaccine production based on a series of tests specified by WHO. Using 'molecular scissors', we clip out the piece of the influenza gene segment responsible for the virus's chicken-killing power and replace it with a piece of gene sequence that is safe. We then replace some of the other gene segments with those from the vaccine strain that we have used previously, which we know provides humans with good protection. Using this strategy we can make 'vaccine seeds' to keep up with the changes that H5N1 and other bird flu viruses undergo in nature. These vaccine seeds are given to companies that make influenza vaccines in case Mother Nature pulls another switch.

A second strategy for dealing with a potential H5N1 pandemic is to produce a medicine that stops the virus from spreading. The main drugs available for this purpose are the anti-neuraminidase drugs described in Chapter 3: Tamiflu (oseltamivir), Relenza (zanamivir), Rapivab (peramivir) and Inavir (laninamivir). They bind to the neuraminidase enzyme on the surface of an influenza virus, thereby preventing the virus from spreading from one cell to another. In this way the drug inhibits the spread of virus between susceptible people. These drugs have been demonstrated to be safe and effective against the circulating H1N1 and H3N2 strains of influenza in humans.

However, laboratory tests of the effectiveness of these drugs in mice and ferrets show that they have some limitations. For example, treatment of mice and ferrets with Tamiflu or the other neuraminidase inhibitors before or within one day of infection with H5N1 saved the animals from death and reduced the amount of H5N1 virus in samples collected from them, but if treatment was delayed until day two, the amount of the virus in the animals didn't drop as much, and by the third day all the animals had died. These results were consistent with those from studies of Tamiflu given to humans infected with any of the circulating human influenza viruses. By three to four days after diagnosis of influenza, treatment had minimal benefit. Tamiflu is a very good drug if given soon enough, but its window of effectiveness is quite small and declines quickly.

There is an urgent need for new drugs for treating influenza, and there are some in the pipeline. A promising new drug being developed in Japan, T-705 (favipiravir), when used together with Tamiflu, can extend the window of effectiveness for treating H5N1 influenza to nearly one week. The use of an old drug called amantadine together with Tamiflu also improves the effectiveness of both. Other new drugs are in the pipeline and are discussed in Chapter 17.

The third option for controlling H5N1 bird flu is to close all live bird markets as soon as the virus is detected. The effectiveness of this strategy is clear from the Hong Kong experience in 1998, when the number of new cases of H5N1 in humans fell from 18 to zero as soon as all LBMs were closed. As a public health scientist, I have to say the optimal choice would be to permanently close all LBMs worldwide, but this would not be easy to achieve. China and some other countries where refrigeration is increasingly available are moving towards closure of LBMs when outbreaks of bird flu occur. However, in countries like Bangladesh, where household refrigeration is often not available, people depend on LBMs for fresh poultry. Moreover, LBMs are so much a part of the culture in many countries that it will take generations for people to accept chilled or frozen poultry and centralised processing. While closing the LBMs has been demonstrated to immediately reduce transmission of H5N1 and H7N9 influenza viruses to humans, centrally processed carcasses are still a source of infectious disease agents including influenza. Cooking poultry and cleaning cutting boards are essential.

The continued operation of LBMs provides influenza viruses with ideal opportunities to continue to mutate, mix and mate, and eventually one will be able to spread human to human. The question of closing LBMs will then be moot, for the horse will have bolted.

In 2009 Mother Nature completely blindsided the influenza experts of the world. Instead of sending another version of H5N1 she sent us an influenza virus that, in all our tests, looked alarmingly like H1N1 – the virus responsible for the 1918 Spanish influenza. It was as if the 1918 experience was about to be repeated, and the virus replanted in the human population for a 90-year anniversary. The virus was quickly dubbed 'swine flu' by the global press, which greatly upset pig farmers in both Mexico and the United States. A belated effort was made by WHO to call the virus H1N1 2009, avoiding the words 'Mexico' and 'swine', both of which implied blame of the country and host in which it was detected, but the informal label stuck.

Although the emergence of the new virus in humans and pigs in Mexico was completely unanticipated, the response to it showed that the WHO influenza network was functioning well. Initial characterisation of the 2009 H1N1 influenza virus, isolated from humans in Mexico, showed that its haemagglutinin was remarkably similar to that of the 1918 Spanish influenza virus. We were of course immediately concerned that the virus might cause disease as severe and widespread as that pandemic. At the time, the outbreak in humans in Mexico seemed mild: the disease lasted two to three days, with only a few severe cases. But we knew how quickly a virus could change and become deadly. Influenza experts around the world felt it was necessary to prepare for the worst-case scenario. Previously arranged strategies for a possible H5N1 influenza outbreak were quickly implemented – vaccine was prepared, and nations were encouraged to stockpile anti-influenza drugs.

Of course the 2009 H1N1 influenza virus did spread out of Mexico, and the resulting disease met all of the WHO's criteria for a pandemic, affecting humans in all countries in the world. Fortunately, the virus did not become extremely deadly. That is not to say that it was a totally 'wimpy' pandemic, as some pundits later observed. It caused an estimated 284,000 fatalities globally. Young people were particularly susceptible, and some ethnic groups, such as First Nations peoples in Canada, were 6.5 times more likely to be admitted to intensive care than the general population.[70] Aboriginal peoples in Australia were also more severely affected, being admitted to intensive care units at a rate 4.5 times higher than other Australians.[71] However, overall, the

2009 H1N1 pandemic was milder than other influenza pandemics. The 2009 H1N1 virus replaced the previously circulating H1N1 strain and has continued to cause seasonal influenza since then.

In the wake of this outbreak, influenza experts in the WHO were taken to task by the Council of Europe for 'mishandling' the pandemic. The council proclaimed that the experts had overestimated the pandemic's likely severity and also might have been compromised by too close an affiliation with industry, recommending the stockpiling of drugs that turned out to be ineffective. They further argued that the vaccines were too little, too late.

WHO took these criticisms very seriously and assembled an international panel of public health officials from several countries to determine whether there had been any wrongdoing.[72] It is true that the pandemic had spread around the world before enough vaccine was available for general use. It is also true that our predictions regarding possible severity had been wrong – because we do not know yet how to scientifically forecast the severity of an influenza epidemic. We therefore erred on the side of caution and of being prepared.

Despite improved ways of rapidly manufacturing influenza vaccine seed strains, it still takes too long to produce a new vaccine, test it for safety and distribute it in sufficient quantities. We cannot do this fast enough to make an impact on the first wave of an influenza pandemic as it sweeps around the world. We cannot treat millions of people with an untested vaccine: it must be tested on a limited number of people first, to ensure that it causes no adverse reactions and that it does induce the intended production of levels of protective antibodies. Since we have now safety tested several H5N1 influenza vaccines, we might be able to speed up any testing of new ones. But producing vaccines to the 2009 H1N1 influenza virus had to start from scratch, and this took about six months. Despite criticism, this vaccine may well have reduced the severity of the outbreak.

The most contentious issue raised by the critics was the allegation that health officials had been influenced by drug manufacturers to recommend stockpiling of anti-influenza drugs. But since those drugs were the best medicine available at the time, this advice was the best that we could give. They are by no means the perfect medicine for influenza, but they have proven benefits. We all know that better drugs are needed, but until they become available, we are stuck with anti-neuraminidase drugs. The idea of a stockpile is to have enough drug prepared so that spread is reduced and treatment is available until a vaccine is prepared, which can take up to six months.

The WHO investigating panel concluded that the organisation had given the best possible advice; that its experts had not been on the take from industry; and that we need a better understanding of influenza severity and how to predict it.

***

The appearance of the H1N1 1918 look-alike influenza virus in 2009 was of great interest to those of us trying to understand where these viruses come from. The unique composition of each new virus allows us to use its individual components to trace its ancestry. We have now traced all of the eight components of that virus back to their origins, and all of them are traceable back to influenza viruses carried in

---

Figure 12.1 The 2009 H1N1 pandemic virus contained gene segments from influenza viruses first detected in pigs in Europe, the US and Mexico. The European swine influenza virus (A) emerged in 1979 from European wild ducks, causing influenza in pigs and occasionally infecting humans. It did not spread from human to human. The American swine influenza virus (B) was first detected in 1998 and was a triple reassortant with two gene segments from American wild ducks (PB2, PA); three gene segments from classic swine influenza virus (NP, M, NS), the descendant of 1918 Spanish influenza; and three gene segments from the circulating human H3N2 influenza virus (PB1, HA, NA). The 2009 H1N1 pandemic influenza virus (C) acquired two gene segments from the European swine influenza virus (NA, M), five gene segments from the American triple reassortant (PB1, PB2, PA, NP, NS) and the haemagglutinin gene from pigs in Mexico.

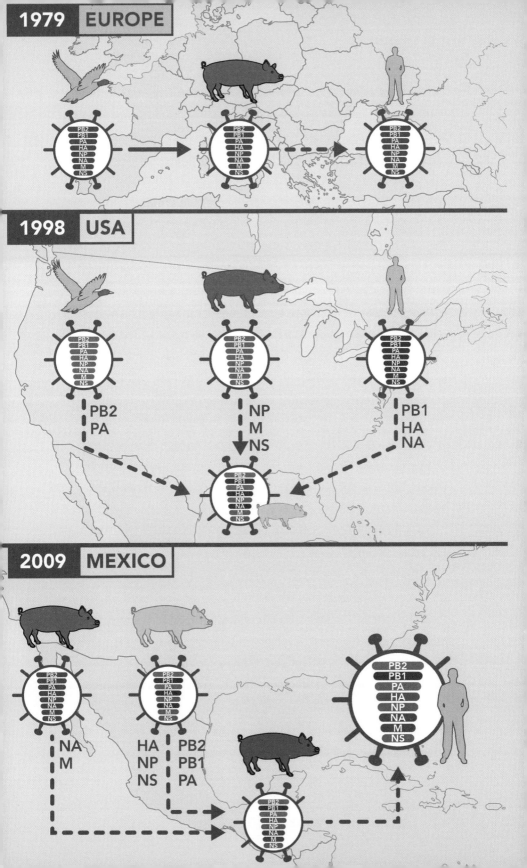

populations of the wild ducks of the world. But they came by different routes, some from the United States and some from Europe (Figure 12.1).

In Europe in 1979 an H1N1 influenza virus from wild aquatic birds spread to pigs. All its components were from wild birds, and this became the dominant influenza virus in pigs in Europe, causing mild respiratory disease. In 1998 a new influenza virus emerged in pigs in the US. This virus caused severe infection in pigs in Texas, Minnesota and Iowa, and replaced the descendants of the 1918 swine influenza virus that had caused influenza in pigs for almost a century. When we looked into its composition, we found it was a 'triple' hybrid virus: it had three parts from human H3N2 influenza viruses (PB1, HA, NA), three components from the classical 1918 influenza virus (NP, M, NS), and two parts from a wild duck influenza virus (PB2, PA).[73]

The H1N1 virus that emerged in Mexico in 2009 contained five components from the triple American swine influenza virus (PB2, PB1, PA, NP, NS), two components from the European swine influenza virus (NA, M), and the haemagglutinin component from pigs in Mexico. We don't know where all these parent viruses met up. The simplest explanation is that European and American pigs were imported into Mexico, where the viruses met and exchanged genetic material.

Although the 2009 H1N1 influenza pandemic was considered relatively mild, it did establish itself in humans worldwide and replaced the H1N1 virus that had been circulating. It also spread to pigs in many places in the world, causing mild disease and also the possibility of more mixing of swine influenza viruses in the future.

After the 2009 pandemic, scientists in Hong Kong published important findings on its origins, as discussed above, based on weekly samples collected from pigs arriving from southern China at a slaughterhouse near Shenzen. They believed the virus had probably been around for some time before it was detected, for little surveillance was done on pigs in Mexico. The study made a major contribution to our understanding of the 2009 H1N1 viruses and was published in the prestigious journal *Nature*.[74]

Shortly after the paper's publication, the Ministry of Agriculture in China called a meeting to discuss this work and compare the results with data collected in China. The government officials clearly seemed to think that Hong Kong scientists were again publishing work without the blessing of the Ministry of the Agriculture. The scientists in the firing line – Gavin Smith, Malik Peiris and Yi Guan – explained that the paper in *Nature* established that the 2009 H1N1 had definitely originated in the Americas and *not* in Asia. Ruffled feathers were thus smoothed.

The detection of both the 1918 and the 2009 H1N1 influenza virus pandemics in the Americas suggests to me that the hemagglutinin genes of both may have originated from viruses in wild aquatic birds in the Americas, while the hemagglutinin, neuraminidase and PB2 genes of the 1957 Asian H2N2 and Hong Kong H3N2 pandemics originated from viruses in wild aquatic birds in Asia.

CHAPTER 13

SARS, AND A SECOND BIRD FLU OUTBREAK

In February 2013 a second bird flu emerged in people and poultry in Shanghai, caused by an influenza virus of the H7 subtype. This was an H7N9 influenza virus, and it caused very mild or unnoticeable disease in chickens but killed about 30 per cent of infected humans. The symptoms in humans were almost identical with those of the H5N1 bird flu: high fever and sore throat, progressing rapidly to pneumonia.[75] While most people infected with H5N1 were otherwise healthy middle-aged women, the people who first contracted H7N9 influenza were older men who had other compromising diseases, such as heart disease, or health issues such as asthma.

The absence of disease or symptoms in poultry in the LBMs at the time meant that humans were again serving as the canaries in the coal mine. The response of Chinese health officials this time was dramatic. Outbreaks of disease in humans and poultry were immediately reported to the WHO, and all available information about the H7N9 influenza virus, including its full genetic code, was published. Chinese health authorities are to be complimented and thanked by the rest of the world for such openness and sharing. The outcome demonstrated the tremendous importance of the 'one world, one health' initiative and was light years ahead of the official response to the 2006 outbreak of severe acute respiratory syndrome (SARS) in China.

It is worth a little detour here from the outbreak of H7N9 to look at SARS, because the infrastructure developed at the University of Hong Kong for responding to H5N1 bird flu served perfectly for the detection of SARS in 2003. SARS is another respiratory disease, caused by a group of viruses related to the coronaviruses, which cause the common cold. SARS is characterized by chills, muscle aches, headaches and loss of appetite, and was initially thought to be caused by the H5N1 bird flu virus. The SARS coronavirus was spread from human to human by respiratory droplets, by faecal contamination and through urine. Mortality was age related, being less than 1 per cent in people under 25 years old and greater than 50 per cent in those aged 65 and older. Originally an animal virus, the virus spread to humans in Guangzhou Province and then to visitors from Hong Kong, who spread the virus to humans in Singapore and Canada. It spread rapidly through hotels and hospitals and showed all the signs of becoming a new pandemic.

Malik Peiris isolated the virus responsible for SARS and identified it as a coronavirus, raising the possibility of making vaccines in the future and developing hygiene strategies for its control.[76] Meanwhile, Yi Guan established that the civet cat (*Paradoxurus hermaphroditus*) in southern China's live animal markets was the intermediate host transmitting the virus to humans.[77] Civet cats were sold in the markets as exotic wildlife for human consumption. They were removed from the markets, and the farms where the animals were bred were closed down. Later it was shown by Kwok Yung Yuen, also from Hong Kong University, that the ultimate source of the SARS virus was the tiny horseshoe bat (*Rhinolophus* species) that is native to Hong Kong. The bat colony was left undisturbed, and people now know the risks of visiting the bat's lodging places.

The rapidity with which the SARS virus had acquired the ability to spread from human to human surprised researchers and was a lesson that influenza virologists must continue to heed. Fortunately an epidemiological study quickly established that hand washing, wearing face masks and practising good hygiene could prevent the spread of the virus. In total, some 8096 people were infected with SARS, and 724 died – 648 in China, 43 in Canada and 33 in Singapore. Once again, containing the outbreak had been hindered by the initial reluctance of health officials in China to share information on the new disease.

***

Now let's turn back to the emergence of H7N9, the second bird flu virus, in Shanghai in 2013. Our knowledge of the role of LBMs in the 1997 H5N1 bird flu led us to suspect that LBMs were the source of the H7N9 virus. Local health officials recommended that LBMs in Shanghai be closed. When that action was taken, the effect was the same as it had been in Hong Kong 16 years earlier: the number of new human influenza cases rapidly fell to zero. It is unclear what happened to all the poultry from the Shanghai LBMs. There are rumours that at least a portion of the H7N9-infected chickens that showed no visible disease were trucked to markets in cities to the south. If this it true, it would explain why the virus spread quickly in cities where the LBMs were not closed.

Laboratory examinations of the virus showed a remarkable similarity to H5N1. Six of the eight components of H7N9 had come from the H9N2 influenza virus. The haemagglutinin surface spike came from a wild duck influenza virus and the neuraminidase from a different wild duck influenza virus (Figure 13.1).

The H9N2 influenza virus was not new, but here it was the enabler, providing H7N9 the ability to spread from poultry to people and to cause severe and even lethal disease. A study of H9N2 viruses in China from 2010 to 2013 showed that they were widespread across most of China and were causing reduced egg production on chicken farms.[78]

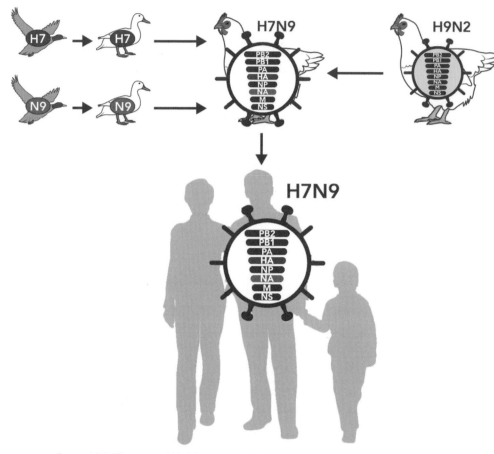

Figure 13.1 The second bird flu virus, H7N9, is a triple reassortant (hybrid) virus. The haemagglutinin (H7) gene segment came from an influenza virus in Asian wild ducks, which spread to domestic ducks; the neuraminidase (N9) gene segments came from a different influenza virus in Asian wild ducks, which also spread to domestic ducks; and the other six segments came from H9N2 in domestic chickens. This new virus, H7N9, began to spread to humans, proving lethal in over 30 per cent of cases.

Back in the early 1990s, poultry vaccines against H9N2 had been developed and administered. Those vaccines were effective at reducing the drop in egg production but also caused the virus to change. As the H9N2 virus changed, new vaccines were made. However, the H9N2 virus eventually reassorted with an H7N9 influenza virus to produce the bird flu virus that was transmitted to humans in 2013.[79]

In the first wave of H7N9 infection in the Shanghai region, 135 people were infected, and 45 died. Studies of the H7N9 influenza virus in the laboratory showed that the virus was picking up features that might allow it to spread from human to human. To determine which of the bird flu viruses (H5N1 or H7N9) had the greatest potential to spread human to human, we did risk-assessment studies in ferrets (the best model we have for testing human transmission risk). Two ferrets were infected (via the nose) with either H5N1 or H7N9, and each was put into a cage containing four healthy ferrets to test for transmission through direct contact. In an adjacent cage, separated by 20 centimetres, were four additional healthy ferrets to test whether the virus was spread by aerosol.

The H5N1 virus spread to all of the ferrets in direct contact with the two infected animals, but not to the ferrets in the adjacent cage. In contrast, the H7N9 virus spread to both the direct-contact ferrets and two of the four ferrets in the adjacent cage, indicating aerosol spread. So the H7N9 influenza virus has greater potential to spread through the air.

After the number of human cases of H7N9 fell to zero, LBMs in Shanghai were reopened, and there were occasional reports of additional human infection. Meanwhile the virus spread to the south of China, and the first human infections were detected in Guangzhou in January 2014. The spread was inevitable, given that affected poultry showed no signs of disease. There was no evidence that migratory birds were involved in the virus's spread, but small domesticated birds like canaries and budgerigars, and small birds such as sparrows were infected experimentally in the high containment laboratory, and they may have spread the virus locally. Since elderly men were the age group initially affected, we wondered if the Chinese tradition of walking and talking with pet birds might have contributed.[80]

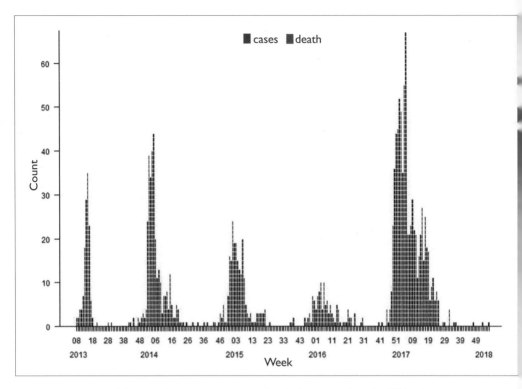

Figure 13.2 A timeline showing the numbers of human cases of H7N9 avian influenza in China since 2013. The numbers peak each year in the winter months. The majority of H7N9 human infections occur through direct contact between humans and poultry, usually in live bird markets. When the LBMs are closed the number of human cases declines dramatically. Over this time there have been a total of 1623 human cases, with 620 deaths. To date the virus has not acquired the ability to spread human to human, but the large increase in the number of cases in 2016–17 is of great concern. Courtesy of World Health Organization

To date, the H7N9 virus has not spread to countries adjacent to China, but humans infected in China have taken the virus to Taiwan. Still, this virus has not acquired the ability to spread human to human – yet! Each winter since 2014, the H7N9 influenza virus has spread from LBMs and caused severe disease and deaths in humans in China. The pattern of this disease has changed, and it infects a wider age range and also otherwise healthy individuals (see Figure 13.2).

***

In early February 2017, when I was in Hong Kong writing about the H7N9 outbreak, there was a larger than usual peak of disease caused by H7N9 influenza virus in humans across China, and the virus underwent a dramatic change. From February 2013 until late 2016, the H7N9 virus had caused imperceptible disease in poultry. Then it became a killer of chickens, like the lethal H5N1 virus. Scientists in China and elsewhere had been expecting this type of change – from benign to killer strain in chickens – because it is one of the known characteristics of the H5 and H7 subtypes of influenza viruses.

We know the exact changes in the H7 spike necessary for it to become a chicken killer and had been watching for this to happen. At the time of writing in 2017, the H7N9 virus was confined to chickens and had not spread to other hosts. Stamping it out, while a huge task, would be merited.

While the H7N9 bird flu virus has flared up every winter in China, its counterpart H5 has also been on the move. A group of highly lethal H5N1 viruses now seems to be permanently entrenched in poultry in many countries and is endemic in China, Vietnam, Indonesia, the Indian subcontinent and Egypt. Back in 2015 a major outbreak in Egypt caused 136 human infections and 39 deaths.

And still this group of viruses continues to change, and many hybrids have emerged. One of these has the ability to spread easily in wild ducks, and in Korea in 2014 it picked up a new neuraminidase spike, becoming an H5N8 influenza virus. This virus literally took wing, and in January–March of 2014 it was detected in wild aquatic birds in Japan. By April–May it had spread to wild aquatic birds in Siberia and Alaska, and by September–October the virus was evident in both wild and domestic poultry in Europe and North America.

This was the first time the dreaded Asian H5 virus had spread to the Americas: the earlier H5N1 had not succeeded in doing so. H5N8 was first detected in a captive-reared gyrfalcon in Washington State.

The virus was identical with the duck H5N8 influenza virus from South Korea and had probably been spread by migratory waterfowl. Immediately after arriving in the Americas, the virus reassorted with influenza viruses already present in wild waterfowl to produce two offspring: an H5N2 and an H5N1 influenza virus. Suddenly there were three deadly H5 influenza viruses in the wild birds in the Washington State area – H5N8, H5N1 and H5N2. The autumn (October–November) southern migration of wild ducks from Alaska and Canada then carried these viruses south, down the Pacific Flyway, and spread all three to commercial poultry flocks in Washington, Idaho, Oregon, and California, resulting in up to 100 per cent mortality in chickens and turkeys (Figure 13.3).

The most devastating and highly contagious virus was the H5N2 strain. In April–May 2015, ducks migrating from Central America to Canada carried the deadly H5N2 virus to the upper Mississippi Valley, an area bristling with poultry farms. Despite warnings about the need for high levels of biosecurity, H5N2 and H5N8 successfully infected over 220 poultry farms. The good news, if there was any, was that no human infections were detected. This may be due to the absence of LBMs in the Midwestern United States. The other possible reason is that H5N8 may have lost some of its ability to spread to humans (obtained from H9N2 viruses) when its genes reassorted with those of the many influenza viruses present in the Americas.

The strategy adopted by agricultural authorities in the US was culling, quarantine, and compensation for the farmers. Over 42 million chickens were culled – about 10 per cent of the total number of chickens in the country – and 7.5 million turkeys – about 3 per cent of the national flock. While this was going on, the H5 influenza viruses were detected in 85 wild birds.

By the summer (July–August) of 2015 the numbers of new outbreaks of H5 influenza viruses in poultry farms had fallen to zero,

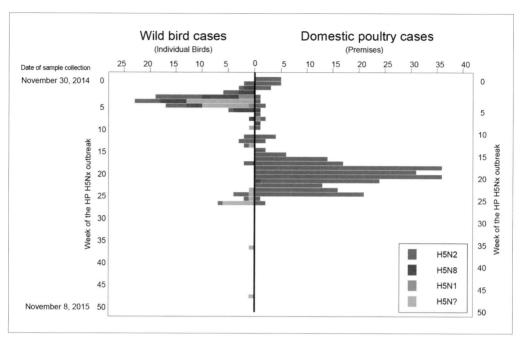

Figure 13.3 Outbreaks of H5Nx influenza in wild and domestic birds in North America. The deadly H5N8 virus on arrival in North America from Korea reassorted with influenza virus in wildfowl and developed H5N1 and H5N2 hybrid viruses, which spread among migratory waterfowl and to domestic poultry farms. The most deadly was H5N2 – more than 42 million chickens and 7.5 million turkeys were culled to contain its spread and stamp it out.

and agricultural authorities were holding their breath while waiting for the migratory ducks from Canada. Would they bring the H5 influenza viruses with them again? Poultry farmers had been begging the Department of Agriculture (USDA) to let them protect their flocks with the poultry vaccine. The USDA had indeed prepared millions of doses of H5 vaccine, but they did not permit the poultry farms to use them (for fear of the viruses becoming endemic – see Chapter 11). The wild ducks arrived on schedule on their way south, but they did not bring the H5 influenza viruses with them. There have been no outbreaks of H5 influenza in poultry farms in North America since

June 2016. Footprints of the H5 viruses (gene sequences like that for the H spike on the H5N2 virus) have been found twice in wild birds in North America, but no live virus has been found.

The apparent disappearance of the lethal H5 influenza viruses from wild aquatic birds is a mystery, and proposed explanations have caused controversy. My research group has been surveying influenza in wild ducks in the US and Canada for over 40 years, and in Alberta, Canada, no lethal H5 or H7 influenza viruses have ever been detected.[81] We believe that wild ducks have an as-yet unknown mechanism to keep the killer H5 and H7 influenza viruses out of the wild duck breeding areas. Yet benign versions of H5 and H7, as well as almost all influenza viruses found anywhere in the world, are regularly found in apparently healthy young ducks.

One possible explanation is that exposure to the vast array of influenza viruses, including non-lethal H5 and H7 viruses, has somehow provided the ducks with herd immunity. Other mechanisms may also be involved, such as the gene in ducks that provides them with inbuilt immunity to influenza. Unfortunately, chickens lost this gene during their evolution from the jungle fowl. However, some scientists disagree with these suggested explanations and believe the lethal H5 virus is still lurking in wild waterfowl. Time will tell. Clearly further scientific research is needed to explain why lethal H5 and H7 influenza viruses are not pathogenic in wild aquatic birds.

Meanwhile, the lethal viruses of the H5 type that persist in Asia have been actively reassorting with influenza viruses in the region to produce an H5N6 influenza virus that caused outbreaks of lethal disease in poultry in China, Myanmar, Taiwan and Vietnam in 2017. These endless changes in the H5 and H7 influenza viruses and their tendency to hybridise and acquire components from other viruses have given rise to grave concerns that eventually they will acquire the ability to spread from human to human. Until very recently, some researchers have believed that since bird flu has been present in the world for 20 years without spreading from human to human, it simply cannot and will not do so. This complacency was shattered when two groups of scientists made an H5N1 bird flu virus that could spread between cages of ferrets and cause severe disease (see Chapter 16).

With all of the active evolution, the numerous subtypes of H5 and H7 and the persistence of these 'hot' influenza viruses in at least four regions of Eurasia, the influenza research community know that it is essential to be prepared and that we urgently need better strategies to deal with the inevitable pandemic in humans.

CHAPTER 14

DIGGING FOR ANSWERS ON THE 1918 SPANISH INFLUENZA

W hat was so special about the 1918 Spanish influenza virus, which killed more people than the two world wars combined? This was a hugely important unanswered question in the 1980s. We needed to get hold of that virus so we could find out its secrets. Unfortunately, since the influenza virus was not isolated until the 1930s, no samples were saved during the 1918 pandemic. Our only hope lay in tissue samples that had been saved from soldiers or influenza patients and were preserved in formalin. These display jars were located in various departments of pathology and in pathological museums. Another possible source of samples was from sufferers who had died in the Arctic regions and were buried in the permafrost. Sixty years later, could we find samples of the 1918 influenza virus in either of these unlikely places?

At scientific meetings in the 1980s, the team at St Jude Children's Research Hospital asked colleagues if they knew of any pathology departments that might have formalin-preserved lung or other tissue from people who had been diagnosed with Spanish influenza. We heard that the US Armed Forces Institute of Pathology in Washington, DC, had a large collection of such tissues from young soldiers who had died in military camps during the peak of the 1918 pandemic. I immediately wrote to Douglas Weir at that institute and proposed a joint study to try to find out why the 1918 influenza virus had been so severe. We knew we would not obtain live virus from the samples, because formalin is also used to kill influenza viruses during the preparation of vaccines. However, we wanted to determine the virus's genetic code, and we were hopeful that the chemicals making up the genetic material of viruses would be sufficiently well preserved for analysis.

We were overjoyed with Weir's immediate and affirmative reply. On 2 February 1990 we received a shipment of formalin-fixed lung samples from nine known victims of 1918 Spanish influenza. Since this was precious material, we developed and then fine-tuned our methods on formalin-fixed lung and respiratory tract tissues of mice and ferrets that had been infected with influenza viruses known to cause severe and lethal disease. Once we were satisfied with our methods, we turned eagerly to the nine human lung samples provided by Weir.

But although the animal tissues had yielded tiny portions of influenza virus genetic code, results from the human tissues were disappointing: we found very little genetic code that we could attribute to influenza. It seemed as if the molecules making up the genetic code of influenza virus had broken apart during their almost 70 years in formalin.

Although our initial foray into this area was frustrating, we were delighted several years later to learn that we had not been barking up the wrong tree. Jeffery Taubenberger, from the Armed Forces Institute of Pathology, had investigated lung tissues from 1918 influenza victims that had been fixed in formalin and then embedded in paraffin blocks for preparation of histological sections. These tissues, which had not been exposed to formalin for as long as the tissues we had analysed, provided the first bits of the genetic code of the 1918 Spanish influenza virus. This groundbreaking work was published in the prestigious journal *Science*.[82]

Now Taubenberger's group had another problem. While the tissue blocks yielded information about the shorter pieces of the influenza virus's genome, our knowledge of the larger pieces of the genome was still incomplete – and they were running out of the lung tissue in the paraffin blocks.

Meanwhile, a team of scientists led by Kirsty Duncan from the University of Windsor, Canada, was attempting to obtain tissue samples of young men who had died of 1918 Spanish influenza en route to the coal mines on Spitsbergen, a Norwegian island approximately a thousand kilometres north of mainland Norway. Each summer the coal mine owners would recruit strong young men in Tromsø, a town on the mainland. The men could earn enough money in one year of mining to buy a small farm, so the competition for positions was fierce.

Duncan found records indicating that seven young men aged 19 to 28 years had been infected while on the ship to Spitsbergen and died of severe influenza shortly after they arrived. They were buried in the churchyard in Longyearbyen, Spitsbergen, on 27 October 1918.[83] Duncan obtained all the necessary permissions to exhume the bodies and collect tissue samples. The international team she assembled comprised geologists, archaeologists, forensic pathologists, physicians and influenza scientists, including myself and other senior influenza virologists from the WHO network.[84] It took a very long time to organise such a complex expedition – six years from inception in 1992 to beginning the exhumation in 1998.

The initial question was whether the crosses in the churchyard cemetery marked the actual graves of the miners, for during World War II the town had suffered extensive bombardment, and most of its structures had been destroyed. To search for burial sites, Duncan's team used ground-penetrating radar that would detect any ground disturbances and their depth. Ground disturbances down to two

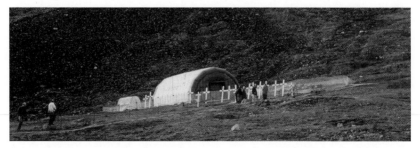

Figure 14.1 The excavation site at the churchyard in Longyearbyen, Spitsbergen, an island off the coast of Norway where seven young men who had died of Spanish influenza were buried in the permafrost.

metres were found for all seven marked graves. Since the active layer in permafrost melts each summer and re-freezes, to a depth of 0.8–1 metre, these findings suggested that the bodies had been frozen in situ for 79 years.

This raised the serious issue of whether live 1918 influenza virus might be released if we indeed found permanently frozen tissues containing the virus. While the scientists agreed that it would be extremely unlikely, none of them could say it was impossible. An already complicated expedition now had to factor in biosafety and biosecurity measures to protect all personnel and the environment.

The work area in the churchyard was entirely covered by an inflatable mobile surgical unit equipped with chemical and decontamination showers, and everyone wore masks and protective clothing. The Longyearbyen locals undoubtedly thought we were a group of mad scientists as they watched several freezers and a shipping container full of assorted equipment being dragged up the hillside (Figure 14.1).[85]

As an additional precaution, we had a supply of the anti-influenza drug Tamiflu on hand in case anyone was exposed during tissue collection. Excavations began, and almost immediately the person digging broke into the first coffin. In keeping with the planned safety measures, he was given Tamiflu right away, but the next morning he complained of severe stomach pain and nausea. Had he released something from the coffin? It seemed highly unlikely, and sure enough he was soon back to normal.

In the event, all our careful planning and safety precautions turned out to be quite unnecessary. The seven coffins were in fact buried in shallow graves, in the active layer of the permafrost, and had been repeatedly frozen and thawed for 79 years. Only the men's skeletons, brain tissue and bone marrow remained, and later analysis of the latter two failed to provide the genetic information we sought. Some of the bodies were wrapped in newspaper, and the dates on the pages coincided with the dates of burial. It seems that the ground-penetrating radar had failed to detect the wooden coffins and the remains, and the ground disturbance two metres down had probably been caused by blasting powder used by the gravediggers to loosen the permafrost.

Although the immaculately planned and executed Spitsbergen expedition came up empty, Taubenberger soon received his much-needed samples – from a completely unexpected source. After publishing his paper on the partial genetic sequence of the 1918 Spanish influenza virus, he received a letter from Johan Hultin, a retired San Francisco physician, asking him if he would like to receive additional tissue from Alaskan victims of the 1918 influenza that were buried in permafrost. Taubenberger could not believe his good fortune, and was delighted when Hultin offered to go to Alaska the following week to obtain the material.

Hultin, it transpired, was driven by a passion similar to Taubenberger's own: to understand why the 1918 influenza had killed so many young people so quickly. Forty-six years earlier Hultin, while a graduate student at Iowa State University, had been part of an expedition to Alaska to isolate the 1918 influenza virus. Back in June 1951 Hultin, Robert McKee and Jack Layton, all scientists from

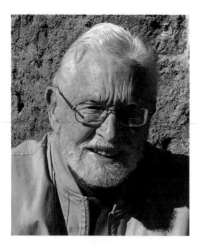

Figure 14.2 Johan Hultin obtained the samples from Brevig Mission that permitted Jeffery Taubenberger to complete the sequence of the 1918 influenza virus.

Iowa State, had flown to Alaska, where they were joined by Otto Geist, a palaeontologist from the University of Alaska, to exhume bodies at Brevig Mission on Seward Peninsula. Samples of lungs were recovered from 1918 victims buried deep in the permafrost. These samples were taken frozen to the university, and Hultin had been sure they would succeed in isolating the influenza virus. But it was not to be. The team completely failed in their attempts to grow the virus in chicken embryos (Figure 14.2).[86]

The 1918 influenza outbreak in this Inuit fishing village is a classic example of just how deadly the 1918 Spanish influenza could be in an isolated community. Hultin told me that in November 1918 a quarantine was in effect in Alaska for all ships with influenza cases on board. The mail ship had stopped at Nome without any known cases of influenza and dropped off mail. But someone on board must have been in the early stages of developing influenza, because the dogsled driver on his 100km drive to the Brevig Mission region was found comatose and later died of severe influenza. He brought the monster virus to the region and at Brevig Mission 72 of the 80 people died. The survivors were mostly children; there were reports of children being found alive in homes where the starving dogs had begun eating the dead parents (Figure 14.3).[87]

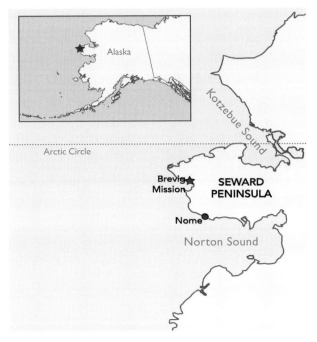

Figure 14.3 A map showing the location of Brevig Mission and Nome in Alaska. On 10 November 1918 the sled-dog musher brought Spanish influenza to the region. Five days later, 72 of the 80 inhabitants of Brevig Mission were dead; remarkably, children survived.

In 1997 Hultin still knew exactly where to find the bodies buried in a mass grave at Brevig Mission. One week after agreeing to obtain samples for Taubenberger, he packed his wife's pruning shears (his only equipment) and flew to Alaska. He met with the village matriarch, who knew that Hultin had previously exhumed bodies, then met the mayor and obtained permission to reopen the mass grave. The village provided four young men to help with the digging.

They dug over two metres deep in the permafrost and located the bodies as expected. From an obese woman in her mid-20s dubbed Lucy, they obtained samples from the optimally frozen lungs, which were filled with blood. They also collected lung samples from less well-preserved bodies. All of the samples were placed in a solution that would kill influenza virus but preserve genetic material (guanidinium thiocyanate). After closing the graves, Hultin built two crosses – one 3.3 metres tall and the other 2.1 metres – to mark the graves and honour the people interred. After returning to San Francisco he divided the samples into several insulated boxes and sent them separately for safety: one by Federal Express, one by the United States Postal Service and one by United Parcel Service. Taubenberger received them all, and the samples from Lucy provided all the material needed for his group to complete the genetic sequence of the entire 1918 Spanish influenza virus.[88]

It was inevitable that comparisons would be made between the successful expedition to Brevig Mission and the unsuccessful expedition to Spitsbergen. In any research project, there is a certain amount of luck involved. At their outset, both expeditions held equal promise. At Brevig Mission the bodies were buried deep in the permafrost, while the Spitsbergen bodies were not. Perhaps the most useful information from the Spitsbergen expedition was that giving Tamiflu on an empty stomach can cause severe stomach ache!

So did finding the entire genetic sequence of the 1918 Spanish influenza virus provide all the answers as to why it was so deadly? Unfortunately the answer is no. The genetic code of the virus on its own was not enough.

CHAPTER 15

RESURRECTING THE 1918 SPANISH INFLUENZA

The lung tissue provided by Johan Hultin, from the woman who had died from the Spanish influenza at Brevig Mission in Alaska in November 1918, yielded the genetic material required to determine the entire genetic code of the 1918 influenza virus.[89] But while it was possible to deduce some features of the 1918 virus from its genetic code – such as its relationship to other influenza viruses – the secret of how it spread so quickly and was so deadly, preferentially killing young adults instead of the very young and elderly, could not be ascertained. To obtain that information it was necessary to remake the 1918 influenza virus from its individual building blocks, as defined by the genetic code. And this mission by Taubenberger's team – to resurrect one of the most deadly infectious disease agents ever recorded – was going to be very controversial (Figure 15.1).

The reaction in public health circles was immediate. A cadre of infectious disease personnel had already contended that the genetic code of the 1918 virus should never have been published, for it provided a blueprint for rebuilding the virus for use as a bioterrorism or biological warfare agent – whose virulence was illustrated by its contribution to the collapse of the German army at the end of World War I. The other issue was the risk of inadvertent release of the virus from the laboratory by infection of a worker, or by the failure of the laboratory's containment measures.

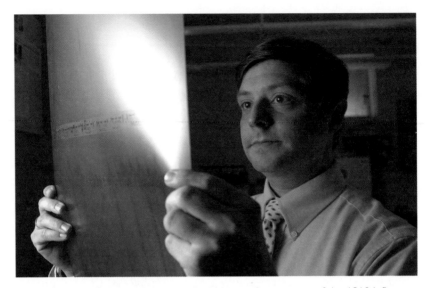

Figure 15.1 Jeffery Taubenberger reading the genetic sequence of the 1918 influenza virus from an autoradiograph film.

These issues had all been carefully considered before publication, by the paper's authors and an advisory committee to the US Secretary of Health and Human Services. (Since this was a national security issue, clearance had to come from the US government.) The advisory committee of the US National Science Advisory Board for Biosafety (NSABB) is made up of a broad range of experts in biological science, public health, biosecurity, law enforcement, national security and biosafety. Weighing the risk that the knowledge of the virus's genetic code could be misused against the benefits of dissemination of the information for the prevention of pandemic influenza, the NSABB unanimously endorsed publishing the research results.

Similarly, after thorough deliberations on the pros and cons of remaking the 1918 influenza virus, the scientific community (including the NSABB) decided that the virus should be remade in high-security laboratories by trained and trusted scientists. Simply put, remaking the virus would reveal why it had become so very deadly, which was vital information if public health defences were to be adequate against future potentially lethal influenza viruses.

Vaccines were on hand to protect the scientists involved, and at least one drug was developed for immediate use. Stringent and specific guidelines were drawn up by the CDC in Atlanta where the work was to be done, to protect the researchers working with these viruses and ensure virus containment. Researchers were required to don air-filtered respirators and protective clothing. No material left the laboratory that was not filtered or autoclaved, including all air, waste and wastewater. Researchers leaving the laboratory first washed down in a chemical shower, then removed the washed protective gear and took a thorough scrub-down shower.

Two kinds of 1918 influenza viruses were prepared: the complete 1918 influenza virus, containing all eight gene segments from the original 1918 influenza virus, and different hybrid viruses, each containing one segment of the 1918 virus and seven segments of a low-pathogenic H1N1 influenza virus. All the viruses were tested for their ability to multiply in mice and ferrets, which they did extremely well and produced high levels of virus, causing high fever and death.

The results were clear: any one of the eight gene segments of the 1918 influenza virus converted a benign virus into a more pathogenic strain. The most deadly virus contained all eight gene segments from the 1918 influenza virus.[90] Each of the 1918 virus's gene segments clearly contained toxic building blocks, but the combination of them all reproduced the 1918 super virus. To determine whether the results from mice and ferrets applied to primates, Kawaoka's group independently remade 1918 influenza virus under the same stringent biosafety conditions and put it into macaque monkeys (*Cynomolgus macaques* [*Macaca fasciculris*]). Every infected animal had to be put down eight days after infection owing to the severity of the disease.[91]

Interestingly, the virus grew to high levels in the respiratory tract of the monkeys (nose, throat, and lungs) but did not spread to the rest of the body.

The research bore out our hypothesis that influenza viruses all come from an avian reservoir: the genetic code indicated that each of the components of the 1918 influenza virus was derived from an ancient avian H1N1 influenza virus that was markedly different from the current H1N1 strains.[92] The severity of the disease caused by the 1918 influenza virus was due to the combined effects of the components of the virus, which attacked multiple parts of the host's defence system.

In response to an infectious agent like an influenza virus, the body has a number of lines of defence. These involve immune cells (the white blood cells), which mount an attack on the invader. The first line of defence is a barrage of chemicals designed to kill the invader, and the first of these are the interferons. These are a large class of cytokine chemicals that interfere with the replication of viruses, further activate the immune response and promote the destruction of virus-infected host cells. Specifically, they inhibit the production of proteins and RNA (the genetic material of influenza viruses) by host cells and the virus alike. Interferons also induce the production of hundreds of other proteins, some of which are involved in further induction of the immune response. As we saw in Chapter 2, the muscle aches and pains associated with influenza infection are caused by these chemicals, which can be extremely toxic if overproduced.

Next, the body begins to produce antibodies that bind tightly to the surface of the invader. These antibodies, together with the many chemicals produced, make it easier for protective scavenging cells (macrophages) to engulf and destroy the invader. The production of an effective number of antibodies takes time – three to five days – explaining why it takes about that long for a healthy person to recover from a mild attack of influenza. After the first encounter with a particular influenza virus, the body remembers how to make that antibody for the rest of its life. This is referred to as 'immunological memory'. The immune systems of people who survived infection with the 1918 influenza virus responded rapidly when they became infected with the 1977 H1N1 Russian flu some 60 years later, and to the 2009 H1N1 pandemic 91 years later.

So why were such a huge number of people killed by the 1918 influenza virus? Research showed that the virus could multiply to very high numbers in infected animals (up to 100 times higher in mice than other H1N1 viruses), and also that it grew extremely well in cultured human lung cells. The high levels of virus multiplication caused extensive damage to the cells lining the respiratory tract – cells that produce surfactants and antiviral chemicals. The high levels of virus also caused the body to respond by producing a 'cytokine storm', a massive release of cytokines that is toxic to the virus but also to the body. So people infected with the 1918 influenza virus died from a combination of high virus loads and high levels of protective but toxic chemicals in their bodies. The lungs of patients filled with fluid, causing their skin to turn blue from lack of oxygen, and the patients finally drowned.

The researchers had discovered that a mild strain of influenza virus is converted into a killer strain when some of the 1918 components are present. These components are the haemagglutinin, the neuraminidase, the PB1 polymerases and the non-structural (NS1) protein. We still do not fully understand their combined effects in making the 1918 influenza virus so deadly, but we have learned that the small NS1 protein and a specific small protein (PB1-F2) coded for by the polymerase PB1 gene somehow block the antiviral response of the host.[93] This reduces the ability of the body to produce interferons. Overall, the 1918 influenza virus is a lethal manipulator. It is like being in a racing car where the safety devices (the foot brake, the handbrake,

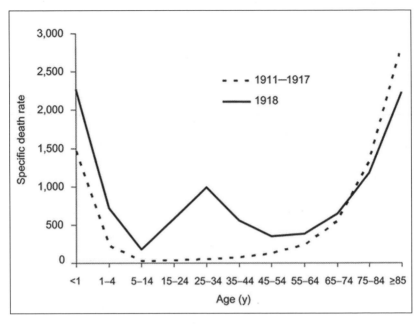

Figure 15.2 The W-shaped mortality curve of the 1918 Spanish influenza. In 1918, Spanish influenza was different from preceding and subsequent influenza pandemics, killing higher numbers in the 25–34 age groups. Reprinted from R.D. Grove and A.M. Hetzel, *Vital Statistics Rates in the United States: 1940–60.* Washington: US Government Printing Office, 1968; and F.E. Linder and R.D. Grove, *Vital Statistics Rates in the United States: 1900–1940.* Washington: US Government Printing Office, 1943

the airbags) are each taken from your control or disabled and the speed increases uncontrollably. The inevitable result is a fatal crash.

Another aspect of the 1918 influenza virus that we don't yet understand is why over half of the people killed were in the 20–40 age group. This resulted in a W-shaped mortality curve, whereas seasonal influenza results in a U-shaped curve, with young children and the elderly being most vulnerable (Figure 15.2). My own opinion is that at the prime of life the body responds to attacks more rapidly and powerfully, so that death resulted from the combination of high levels of destructive virus and the production of very high levels of toxic chemicals to fight the virus. Another hypothesis is that the people in the 20–40 age group who died in 1918 had been infected with the Russian flu of 1890–91 (H3Nx) in childhood. When they were exposed to an identical epitope on the 1918 virus their immune system went into overdrive, resulting in a cytokine storm and death.[94] I hope this hypothesis does not hold up, for it would not bode well for the universal vaccine to influenza that is under intense study.

Many people who survived the virus's initial attack in 1918 later died of bacterial pneumonia. Since there were no antibiotics available then, bacterial infection accounted for many of the total deaths. In 1918 it was believed that influenza was caused by a bacterium called *Haemophilus influenzae* (Chapter 1) but subsequent studies showed that the causative agent was a virus. The combined infection of the 1918 influenza virus and the bacterial infection proved deadly, as the virus manipulated and suppressed the body's defences, allowing bacterial pneumonia to rage with impunity.

There is considerable controversy about whether certain nervous system disorders are linked to survival of the 1918 influenza virus. There was an increased incidence of Parkinson's disease and 'sleeping sickness' (encephalitis lethargica) after the 1918 pandemic, and links between these conditions and infection with the influenza virus were reported in the scientific literature in 1982.[95] However, the many experiments with reconstructed 1918 influenza virus in mice, ferrets and monkeys all showed that the virus infected only the respiratory tract. There was no evidence that the reconstructed 1918 influenza viruses spread through the bloodstream to other organs, including the brain.[96]

That being said, I hasten to add that mice, ferrets and monkeys are not humans, and that only a relatively small number of animals has been examined, compared with the millions of humans affected by influenza in 1918. I suggest that in a very small number of humans, influenza viruses do spread to the brain and cause later neurological effects. The relevant genetic differences in humans are not fully understood. We know that some strains of H5N1 can spread to the brains of mice and that these mice show changes in their brains exactly like brain changes associated with Parkinson's in humans.[97] Such effects might indeed explain the actions of President Woodrow Wilson, who was infected with the deadly strain of 1918 influenza during the peace talks in Paris, suffered severe mental problems and ended up capitulating to French demands to humiliate and destroy Germany.

We have discovered a lot by remaking the 1918 influenza virus, but we also know there is still much research to be done. We need to produce medicines that inhibit the ability of such viruses from multiplying, spreading rapidly and manipulating the body's defence mechanisms. We also need to develop strategies to prevent our bodies from overproducing their own protective, yet toxic, chemicals.

The elucidation of the genetic code of the 1918 influenza virus from tiny fragments of the virus's genome in a piece of lung tissue embedded in a paraffin block from an infected soldier – and the lung tissue of an infected person from the permafrost in Alaska – was a masterpiece of scientific detective work. This work by Jeffery Taubenberger and his team was like piecing together a novel from multiple copies of the book that had been put through a shredder. The pieces of overlapping 'text' were teased out of the jumble until reproducible, overlapping sentences emerged. This mammoth decoding task took nine years and provided the key to our present understanding of the deadly nature of the Spanish influenza virus.[98]

CHAPTER 16

OPENING PANDORA'S BOX

The work of resurrecting the 1918 Spanish influenza virus demonstrated that scientists now have hitherto-unimagined power. We can change a virus's RNA to make the virus multiply, or turn a non-pathogenic influenza virus (such as a virus from migratory birds) into one that can spread and kill. But should we? Is this not akin to opening Pandora's box and letting the evil out?

The 1918 Spanish flu virus is considered to be one of the deadliest infectious agents in the history of mankind. It infected at least 30 per cent of humans globally and killed perhaps 5 per cent of those people. At the peak of the pandemic, cities throughout the world struggled to function and to pick up the dead. So, think what might occur if either of the two bird flus described in previous chapters developed the ability to spread from human to human. H5N1 kills about 60 per cent of humans infected, and H7N9 kills about 30 per cent of those infected.

Twenty years after it was first detected in Hong Kong, H5N1, the first bird flu virus, is still present in domestic poultry in China, Vietnam, Indonesia, Cambodia, Bangladesh and Egypt and periodically spreads to humans, mainly through live bird markets, causing sporadic outbreaks. The second bird flu virus, H7N9, first detected in Shanghai in 2013, is still confined to China. At the time of writing, H5N1 has infected 859 people, with 453 deaths; H7N9 has infected 1532 people, with 581 deaths. The latter virus possesses properties that might make it more likely than H5N1 to acquire the ability to transmit from human to human. To date, thankfully, it has not done so.

These high death rates in humans are difficult to interpret because so many people work in the poultry industry without apparently being infected. The key question here, then, is whether some people are especially susceptible to bird flu viruses. Is there a genetic susceptibility of a section of the human population? The question is not yet answered, but with more and more human genome analysis under way, it may soon be. I believe we will find that there are people who are genetically more susceptible to bird flu, but that the eternally mutating and reassorting influenza virus will potentially circumvent everyone's defence mechanisms and, as in 1918, most people will become susceptible.

However, complacency about bird flu viruses and their supposed inability to spread from human to human is on the rise. 'Since it hasn't happened in 20 years, it is unlikely to occur' is the general attitude. Some scientists also point out that in the known history of influenza, only three subtypes of influenza viruses – H1, H2 and H3 – have caused pandemics in humans, and that the problematic influenza waves seem to cycle through these three groups, so we don't need to worry about any others.

Concerned by this complacency about the possible dangers of bird flu to humans, in 2006 the US National Institutes of Health Blue Ribbon Panel on Influenza Research and the WHO Influenza Research Agenda embarked on an investigation to find out whether the H5N1 virus could ever acquire the ability to spread from human to human. Their research would mean deliberately modifying the virus so that it would gain the ability to spread from animal to animal.

Such experiments are referred to as 'gain of function' experiments. The specific goal was to create an H5N1 influenza virus that could spread between separated cages of ferrets.

Two groups of scientists set to work. One group, at the Erasmus Medical Centre in Rotterdam in the Netherlands, was led by Ron Fouchier; the other, at the University of Wisconsin, was led by Yoshihiro Kawaoka. The Fouchier group modified an avian H5N1 influenza virus isolated from a human infected in Indonesia in 2005 to make it transmissible between ferrets. They first caused the RNA of the virus to change by a process known as site-directed mutagenesis: they changed the virus's genetic code so that it could multiply in mammals. Then they infected the ferrets through the nose with the virus. On the fourth day after infection, the virus from the first ferret was used to directly infect a second ferret, and this process was repeated 10 times (referred to as passages). In the end, the resulting virus spread by aerosol between ferrets in different cages.

Meanwhile, the Kawaoka group used a hybrid virus that contained the haemagglutinin protein of an H5N1 influenza virus isolated from a human infected with H5N1 bird flu in Vietnam in 2004, combined with seven gene segments from the H1N1 virus that caused the 2009 human pandemic. They first introduced random mutations into the genetic segments coding for the H5 component, then created the hybrid virus and finally infected the ferrets, again via the nose. This H5N1 hybrid virus was also shown to be transmissible by aerosol between ferrets in separate cages.

Each of these studies was carried out in high-security facilities under the same stringent guidelines and safeguards required for the work on resurrecting the 1918 influenza virus. The scientists involved were likewise vaccinated against the H5N1 virus and wore full protective gear.

These two studies clearly demonstrated that the H5N1 influenza viruses can acquire the ability to spread between ferrets. It is highly probable that such viruses would also be transmissible from human to human. The studies also showed that a small number of changes, perhaps as few as five, would permit the viruses to spread. It was apparent that transmissibility could come about either by changing an avian H5N1 influenza virus or by mixing genes from different viruses and producing hybrid H5N1 viruses.

This information sheds light on how pandemic influenza viruses might be generated in nature. The highly lethal 1918 Spanish influenza viruses may have been generated by exposure to the chemical agents used during World War I. Perhaps deadly mustard gas caused the key mutational changes in the original virus. High troop concentrations in the trenches would have set the scene for human-to-human transmission of the mutated virus. Repeated transmission from human to human is what the Fouchier group modelled with its 10 passages of their mutated virus in ferrets.

While the 1918 pandemic virus probably involved the transmission of a purely avian influenza virus to humans, subsequent pandemics – including the H2N2 Asian pandemic of 1957, the H3N2 Hong Kong pandemic of 1968 and the H1N1 pandemic of 2009 – all involved hybrid viruses that possessed novel haemagglutinin and neuraminidase components from an avian source but retained some gene segments from 1918 influenza viruses. The experiments by the Kawaoka group with the H5N1 virus adapted to ferrets mimics the genesis of these particular pandemic viruses.

When knowledge of the generation of a ferret-transmissible H5N1 became known to the scientific community, a firestorm erupted. On Monday, 12 September 2011, I had breakfast with Fouchier at the fourth European influenza conference for scientists in Malta. During the meal, he told me of their extremely interesting results and said he

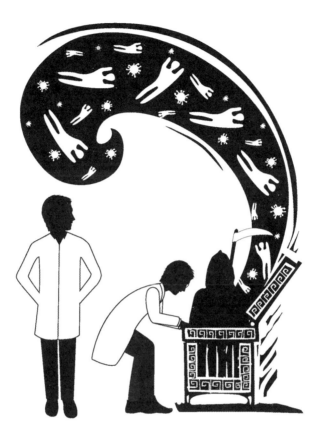

Figure 16.1 Opening Pandora's box …
Cartoon prepared by Elizabeth Stevens, Department of Biomedical Communications, St Jude Children's Research Hospital, Memphis

would present them in his keynote address that morning. I realised the huge impact the findings would have, and I remember sitting with Peter Doherty, the Nobel laureate immunologist, in the session and saying to him that the public would accuse scientists of having opened Pandora's box (Figure 16.1).

Unfortunately some people got the idea from Fouchier's presentation that the H5N1 virus not only was spread from ferret to ferret but that it had killed the ferrets. This was incorrect. The ferrets were killed in a separate study, when the H5N1 virus was injected directly into their windpipe (trachea). But the excitable science journalists in the audience associated transmissibility with death, considerably raising the level of public concern about generating such deadly viruses, and leading to articles in major newspapers about scientists engineering bioterrorism agents. The public firestorm was fuelling itself.

The results from studies by the Kawaoka group on ferret-transmissible H5N1 influenza viruses were released after they had been sent to scientific journals for publication. The studies confirmed the work of the Fouchier group: with only a small number of changes in the haemagglutinin component, H5N1 influenza viruses could be produced that spread from ferret to ferret. The Kawaoka group also pointed out that the changes required to make H5N1 transmissible were already present in the various H5N1 viruses that were causing disease in poultry and humans, but not all changes were present in the same virus. The question was, and is, how long will it take Mother Nature to put these five changes needed into the correct orientation in the same virus? While these studies raise legitimate concerns about bioterrorism and the accidental escape of killer viruses, they also alert the world that as long as these bird flu viruses are circulating, sooner or later nature will deal a deadly hand.

These two studies raised enormously important issues for the scientific community to consider. Is it appropriate to conduct this research, let alone publish the findings? In response to the public outcry, scientists working on influenza viruses called a voluntary moratorium on all gain-of-function studies on emerging viruses in 2011. The studies were considered 'dual use research of concern' (DURC). This meant that, on one hand, the studies on the production of ferret-transmissible H5N1 viruses had clear benefits to knowledge, such as improving our understanding of the potential for the virus to spread in humans and cause a pandemic, and they were important to the development of vaccines and antiviral medicines. But on the other hand, they raised serious concerns about the possibility of accidental release of the H5N1 viruses and of their nefarious use as a bioterrorism agent. The argument was that the blueprint for producing such a terrifying agent should not be published.

It was a difficult time for the NSABB for deciding whether to publish the scientific papers by the Fouchier and Kawaoka groups. They were strongly lobbied from both sides. The committee first erred on the side of caution and opted to publish them only after the removal of key information about the methods used, but after numerous meetings and consultations the papers were published in their entirety in leading journals – the Fouchier group's report in *Science*,[99] and the Kawaoka group's report in *Nature*.[100] The papers emphasised the high levels of biosafety and biosecurity enforced and the fact that the H5N1 influenza viruses containing the dangerous building blocks were already circulating in various parts in the world; the greatest threat was from Mother Nature.

After the publication of these papers, additional biosafety precautions were mandated, and the voluntary moratorium on gain-of-function studies was lifted in 2013. Several more scientific papers were published describing experiments increasing the biological activity of influenza viruses (i.e. gain of function), giving rise to more discussion of whether experiments with viruses like H5N1 should be permanently banned. Then two serious violations of biosecurity at the CDC in Atlanta – one involving the release of anthrax spores and a second involving the sending of an influenza virus culture contaminated with live H5N1 virus to another laboratory – set off alarm bells in the press and among public health scientists. Although neither of these events resulted in human infection or spread of the agents, they served as a wake-up call and pointed to a need for additional levels of control.

These incidents underlined that even the regulators of biosecurity and biosafety can make mistakes, and that many levels of security are necessary. A group of 18 leading scientists – the Cambridge Working Group – called for an immediate cessation of all gain-of-function studies and a thorough examination of all aspects of the control and regulation of dangerous infections like H5N1 influenza virus agents, known as select agents. The National Institutes of Health in the US immediately reimposed the moratorium on gain-of-function research, and the White House Office of Science and Technology Policy requested that the National Academy of Sciences, Engineering and Medicine and the NSABB consider all aspects of the problem.

Those bodies were tasked with organising two open discussions between scientists and the general public on the risks and benefits of gain-of-function research. The issue was to be fully debated, and participants were to make recommendations on the way forward. In recognition of the global significance of the issue, the leading scientific organisations from around the world were involved. I was one of many participants at both symposia. The first took place in December 2014, the second in March 2016. The process has been extremely thorough and detailed, involving participants from many countries in which the biological research under way could result in a disease agent's gaining function.

It is worth considering the term 'gain of function', for it is often thought to refer only to functions that are of high risk to society, such as person-to-person transmissibility in the case of a virus. But the term also refers to highly desirable functions needed for the production of influenza vaccine. For example, when first isolated from humans, influenza viruses often grow poorly in chicken embryos. To make a virus multiply to the levels we need for large-scale vaccine production, we first make a hybrid virus that includes gene segments from known and safe, high-growing vaccine strains. We then 'passage' the hybrid viruses in the chicken embryo, creating far more virus. These studies clearly involve gain of function, but they do not pose a risk. The problem is with DURC gains of function, those that carry both scientific benefits and public health risks.

On 19 December 2017 the US National Institutes of Health lifted the funding pause on gain-of-function experiments involving influenza, SARS and Middle East Respiratory Syndrome that was implemented in October 2014. They also provided recommendations for the evaluation and oversight of the proposed gain-of-function research of concern, recommended by the NSABB. Before any research begins, the project must be assessed to determine whether it is in the DURC category. This involves a rigorous three-stage review and assessment. If the research is found to be of concern, it goes to a final panel that considers whether the proposed research meets all the guidelines of risk mitigation; only if it does is the study approved, and even then it must undergo national inspections. While the proposed recommendations apply to all research funded by the United States government they are not enforceable for privately funded research or in other countries. The hope is that involving the general public as well as international organisations will lead to similar guidelines being adopted.

These multiple levels of review minimise risk levels. Regardless, nothing in life is totally risk free. Scientists dealing with such issues must police themselves closely to make sure they follow the guidelines, cut no corners and institute buddy systems by which scientists supervise one another's work. It is still unresolved who sent anthrax spores by mail to United States news offices and two United States senators, killing five people and injuring 17 others beginning on 18 September 2001. A scientist who worked at the biodefense laboratories at Fort Detrick was suspected and he committed suicide in July 2008.

The motive was never resolved but this event amply illustrates the need for a buddy system to reduce such risks.

The only way to reduce the risk to near zero would be to recommend indefinitely retaining the gain-of-function moratorium on such studies. The reader may agree wholeheartedly with this solution to the problem, but in fact even this would not completely eliminate the risk. Pandora's box is already open, and not every scientist in the world has to abide by the recommendations of United States scientific bodies.

Additionally, Mother Nature is doing her best to keep us very concerned about the spread of the second bird flu (H7N9) in China. There have been over 1000 reported human infections since the first one in 2013, with approximately 30 per cent of infected people now dead. The use of vaccine to H7N9 influenza in poultry in 2018 has dramatically reduced the number of human cases and the incidence of disease in poultry. To date this virus has not spread out of China, which may be explained by its absence in domestic and wild ducks. However, as long as the Asian H5Nx and H7Nx viruses continue to circulate they are a threat to animal and human health. Additional research is urgently needed to prepare new medicines and better vaccines. We cannot achieve this without continued gain-of-function studies, conducted in full compliance with all the guidelines.

CHAPTER 17

LOOKING TO THE FUTURE: ARE WE BETTER PREPARED?

The question uppermost in my mind as we look at the past 100 years of influenza pandemics, epidemics and control strategies is whether another pandemic like the 1918 Spanish influenza, with such a deadly and disruptive impact on society, is possible. The answer is yes: it is not only possible, it is just a matter of time.

At the time of writing, it was evident that as long as the second bird flu virus – the H7N9 strain – continues to circulate in the domestic poultry of China, it will continue to be a pandemic threat. Let us suppose that H7N9 acquires human-to-human transmissibility and retains its lethal nature for humans, causing a 30 per cent or higher mortality rate. How well prepared are we to deal with such an event? Certainly better than people were in 1918, but not as well as we need to be.

Immediate strategies to deal with the problem would include:

1. Administering stockpiled anti-influenza medicines known as neuraminidase (N) inhibitors. As mentioned earlier, to be effective, these drugs must be administered within two to three days of a person's becoming infected.

2. Vaccinating to protect the population against the virus. Unfortunately, any prepared and stockpiled vaccines against H7N9 would probably be outdated, because all viruses continue to change. Those vaccines might well prevent death but might not protect

against infection. It would be essential to make a new H7N9 vaccine as quickly as possible.

3. Using stockpiled universal anti-influenza antibody. This antibody is still at the experimental stage of development. It protects animals against all known influenza viruses and, most importantly, the protection lasts for longer after infection than that of the neuraminidase drugs. It would be a gigantic undertaking to get enough of such an antibody stockpiled, but it must be considered.

4. Using universal influenza vaccine on humans worldwide once the vaccine has been thoroughly safety tested. This would be the best strategy, but it will not be feasible until sometime in the future, perhaps 10 years or more, because the initial tests of universal vaccines in humans has just begun.

We would definitely handle a pandemic now better than the world could in 1918, but would we do any better than we did in controlling the relatively rather mild H1N1 pandemic of 2009, when close to 300,000 people perished? A reality check suggests that we are marginally better prepared now, but that we could not stop an influenza pandemic. Millions of people would die before we could bring it under control or modify its effect.

From where might such a pandemic spring? Since the mid-1990s, influenza has occurred more and more frequently in intermediate hosts, including pigs and poultry. The viruses of greatest concern are the H2, H5, H7 and H9 subtypes. The H2 group caused a human influenza pandemic from 1957 to 1968. The H5, H7 and H9 influenza viruses have periodically spread to humans, causing disease, but have not yet caused pandemics. The H5N1 viruses have become established in the domestic poultry of many countries, including China, Indonesia, Vietnam, Bangladesh and Egypt. It is noteworthy that the H5 group of highly pathogenic influenza viruses were never reported in humans before the mid-1990s; now they are found in humans in several countries every year.

It could be argued that the apparent increased incidence of influenza in pigs and poultry is in fact due to more intense surveillance. It is true that influenza surveillance in these animals has vastly improved since the mid-1990s, but that is not the only reason for the increase. Another reason is that the global populations of intermediary hosts for influenza – ducks, chickens and pigs – have grown to meet increasing demand for protein as the world population rises. The Food and Agriculture Organization of the United Nations estimates that the global population of chickens increased more than sixfold between 1961 and 2013, while domestic ducks increased fivefold, pigs more than doubled and the human population did the same. The continued presence of highly pathogenic H5N1 and H7N9 and the less pathogenic H7N9 and H9N2, which periodically spread to humans in live bird markets, is of continuing concern.

Since we know that influenza pandemics originate from the aquatic bird reservoirs of the world and that the viruses spread through live poultry markets, or via pigs, to humans, it makes sense to attempt to prevent that initial spread. Prevention would seem to be the best policy. The closure of all the LBMs in Hong Kong in 1997 immediately interrupted the spread of H5N1 to humans. After the LBMs were reopened, the virus returned. After the emergence of the second bird flu (H7N9) in Shanghai in 2013, the number of human cases similarly fell quickly after the LBMs were closed.

From a public health perspective, permanently closing LBMs worldwide makes good sense. And it will be too late to do so *after* any of the bird flu viruses (H2, H5, H7, H9) have acquired the ability to spread from human to human. However, many countries are highly dependent on these markets. Closing them would be problematic in nations where household refrigeration is limited; LBMs are traditionally the safest way for consumers to obtain fresh meat.

The experience in Hong Kong has shown that the situation can change over time, however. There, the number of LBMs has fallen from over 1000 in 1997 to 132 in 2017, and people no longer depend completely on such markets. While the older members of society in Hong Kong firmly believe that live-bought chicken tastes much better than the frozen equivalent, the younger generation is moving to consumption of refrigerated or frozen chicken. One goal would be to encourage other countries to rely less on LBMs. Another goal should be to encourage countries like China and the US, where alternatives are plentiful, to begin working towards permanent closure of their LBMs for poultry.

Another way to help prevent the spread of influenza viruses to humans is to develop poultry and pigs that are resistant to influenza. We know that some animals (such as sheep) and some duck breeds (such as mallards) are naturally resistant. In Chapter 11 we saw that these ducks showed no disease when infected with a strain of H5N1 bird flu that kills 100 per cent of infected chickens and turkeys.

We now know that during the evolution of the domestic chicken from the jungle fowl, the gene for interferon, the first line of defence against influenza, was lost. All ducks have this gene. If we were to transfer this duck gene (RIG-I) to chickens, then chickens would probably not be killed by the H5N1 virus. The downside of course would be that the chicken would then become the ultimate Trojan horse in the spread of influenza – a carrier with no visible signs!

The gene for interferon is only one of many providing some protection. A better strategy would be to make chickens (and/or pigs) completely resistant to influenza. As we define all the genes that make a sheep naturally resistant to influenza, these genes could be transferred to chickens and/or pigs. This in turn of course raises the issue of the ethics – along with the risks and benefits – of the genetic engineering of animals and the manipulation of human genes. These decisions are for the future, and the possibility of influenza-resistant animals is part of that future.

Universal vaccines are much closer to being realised than influenza-resistant pigs and poultry. Scientists have discovered that all subtypes of influenza A viruses contain common or universal parts of the haemagglutinin (H) component. Figure 2.2 in Chapter 2 of the H component is useful here: the common region of this club-shaped spike would be the stalk (the head, sitting on top of the stalk, projects outside the virus). Universal antibodies have been prepared that attach to these common regions and halt infection by all subtypes of influenza viruses. The difficulty is that lower animals and humans make the vast majority of their protective antibodies to attach to the head of the club. Only a tiny proportion of antibodies are made for the common regions. Although scientists have successfully cultured generations of cells that produce antibodies to these common regions, those cell lines are extremely rare. However, many pharmaceutical companies have prepared universal antibodies and have begun to market them. While these will be useful for treating severe cases of influenza infection in humans, there are not enough available to control a rapidly spreading influenza pandemic.

We urgently need a universal vaccine, but this is still a pipe dream. The challenge is to make a vaccine that will persuade the human body to preferentially make antibodies to the stalk of the H spike. Many approaches are being tested in animals and humans, each attempting to direct the body's immune response to these common regions. The approaches include cutting off the head of the H spike and putting on different heads, using only the stalk region to make a vaccine and creating a length of DNA that specifies the common region and then priming the human body with a DNA-based vaccine.

Eventually one or more of these strategies will be shown to provide universal protection to all influenza viruses. The next challenges will be to determine and then demonstrate that these vaccines are safe and have no downside, such as making the virus more easily taken into cells. Once all the safety and effectiveness goals are achieved, influenza scientists' dream of a universal vaccine may well be realised.

This all sounds like an extremely protracted undertaking, but our experience from the 2013 bird flu (caused by the H7N9 virus) suggests that it may not necessarily be. After Chinese scientists published the virus's complete genetic code, commercial companies immediately started to make the haemagglutinin and neuraminidase surface components of the influenza virus using the genetic information. As a result, a DNA vaccine to the virus was available within weeks. This effort demonstrated the wisdom of sharing information.

Unfortunately, there are very few anti-influenza drugs available that make much impact. Currently we have one ancient family of 'plug drugs' (amantadine and rimantadine), which plug up the tiny pipeline into the virus's core – the M2 protein. While they do work, influenza viruses rapidly become resistant to them, and they are rarely used. The more effective family of drugs targets the neuraminidase component (Tamiflu, Relenza, Rapivab and Inavir). These drugs block the enzyme so the virus remains stuck to the host cell and cannot spread. They are very effective if administered immediately a person becomes infected but are not helpful after about two days. However, they are the best we have so far.

Two new drugs, T-705 (favipiravir) and Baloxavir marboxil (Xofluza), are showing considerable promise for treatment of influenza. These drugs target different components of the polymerase complex. Both drugs are approved for human use in Japan: T-705 was approved for emergency use against oseltamivir (Tamiflu) resistant viruses in 2014 and Xofluza was approved for treatment of influenza in February 2018. T-705 is what we call a nucleotide analogue – it looks like one of the building blocks of a virus genome, but when incorporated into the virus's RNA it makes it non-functional. Xofluza binds to a pocket in the PA protein and blocks its function in replication. A single oral dose of this drug is sufficient to treat influenza infection in humans, making it very convenient.

Each of these drugs targets a different vital pathway in the replication of an influenza virus. Used in combination with a neuraminidase inhibitor (Tamiflu), they would have real impact on reducing the spread of an influenza pandemic. Many other anti-influenza drugs are also under development, so a well-equipped drug toolkit is in the pipeline. And we are already much better off than the world population in 1918.

Another advantage we have today is antibiotics. Bacterial pneumonia, which was responsible for many of the deaths in the 1918 Spanish influenza pandemic, can now be treated with antibiotics, and pneumococcal vaccines can be used to prevent infection caused by the bacterium *Streptococcus pneumoniae*. But there are two difficulties: the population's increasing resistance to antibiotics, and the fact that not enough people are vaccinated against bacterial infection. The elderly are at particular risk and should receive both the pneumonia and yearly influenza vaccines. As a senior myself, I strongly recommend both to all my contemporaries – the benefits are scientifically proven and the risks are extremely low.

A question I am frequently asked is, will we be able to predict the next influenza pandemic? Currently, we cannot do so; however, I am an optimist. I remember the weather forecasts of 70 years ago – they were often wrong and rarely even predicted major storms. Forecasters simply did not have the information they needed. Fast forward to today, when weather forecasts are much more precise and often even correct!

When the influenza forecasters are able to get information of equivalent quality and quantity, I am optimistic that they will be able to predict the next influenza epidemic or pandemic. But there is so much more we need to know. At one point we thought that finding the genetic code of the influenza virus would give us the answer. Well, it gave us some information, but to find the full answer we had to remake the virus. This process in turn provided valuable information on the many techniques the virus uses to circumvent the defence mechanisms of the human body. We discovered that because the 1918 virus made such vast amounts of virus in the host's body, the body overproduced its own toxic protective chemicals, thus turning the guns on itself. To fully understand the mechanisms involved there, we need to know the full genetic code of humans and the myriad different pathways of interplay between it and the virus. And of course many other species are involved, adding complexity to the issue.

While pandemic influenza has been the central theme of this book, seasonal influenza is also of serious concern. Cumulatively seasonal influenza kills more people globally than pandemics (with the exception of 1918). The 2017–18 seasonal outbreaks of influenza in Britain and the US illustrate the point. These outbreaks were dominated by an H3N2 influenza virus that was dubbed 'Aussie flu' by the British press. Genetically the virus could be traced back to Australia from Britain and the US. The H3N2 virus was similar to the virus from the previous season, but the severity of the disease was greatly increased. It killed over 100 children in the US and filled hospitals. The recommended vaccine provided limited protection (10–30 per cent efficacy). Antigenically the H3N2 virus was similar to the virus from the previous season, but the severity was greatly increased. Much better vaccines are urgently needed, and we need to understand why severity can vary so greatly and how to treat severe cases.

It is sobering to realise that, after nearly 100 years of studying the 1918 influenza, we still do not know precisely why the virus was such a killer; nor are we significantly better prepared to deal with a repeat event. We have made huge advances in our understanding, and in the development of medicines and vaccines, but we are not there yet.

It is a very exciting time in biological sciences – we have the power to play God, to make changes in the genetic codes of viruses, animals and humans and help make better medicines, vaccines and resistant animals. The challenge will be to regulate ourselves sufficiently to protect society from mistakes but not so far as to stifle our ability to generate scientific knowledge. For nature will eventually again challenge mankind with an equivalent of the 1918 influenza virus. We need to be careful, but we also need to be prepared.

GLOSSARY

aerosol – Tiny airborne particles, such as viral particles ejected from the body by sneezing, which can spread influenza.

agglutination – The sticking together of small particles, such as red blood cells, to make a visible clump.

antigenic variation – The mechanism by which an infectious agent alters its surface proteins in order to evade a host immune response.

autoclave – A device for sterilising scientific equipment and materials with a combination of heat and high atmospheric pressure.

backbone light chain – The chain of amino acids that makes up the stalk of the major spike protein on the surface of the influenza virus.

chemokines – A family of small *cytokines* that attracts *phagocytes* and cells involved in induction of immunity to the site of infection and provides the first lines of defence from infection with influenza.

cloaca – The cavity near the anus of birds and reptiles that collects intestinal and urinary tract waste, and in females serves as a depository of sperm. Swabs from birds' cloacas can detect influenza virus infection.

coronavirus – A family of viruses different from influenza that can cause respiratory tract infection with high fever and pneumonia. Examples are the common cold virus and *SARS*.

cyclotron – A large atomic device for accelerating charged atomic particles in a magnetic field. The beam of charged particles can be used to determine the structure of molecules, including parts of influenza viruses.

cytokines – Small protein molecules that provide the first line of defence against disease agents. They signal infection to the cells inducing antibodies and cellular immunity.

cytokine storm – An overproduction of *cytokines* that can be fatal. This contributed to fatalities from bird flu (H5N1) and 1918 Spanish influenza.

DNA (deoxyribonucleic acid) – The helical molecule that carries the genetic information of an organism and is replicated during cell reproduction.

enzyme – A catalyst that speeds up a chemical reaction without itself being changed.

epidemic – A contagious disease that spreads rapidly and widely, e.g. influenza.

fowl plague – A lethal disease of poultry caused by the highly *pathogenic* H5 and H7 influenza viruses. It spreads throughout the bird's body, causing haemorrhages in all organs.

genetic drift – Random changes in genetic information (mutations). Genetic drift causes changes in the H and N surface spikes of influenza viruses that require annual changes to flu vaccines.

genetic shift – In influenza viruses, a complete change of the *haemagglutinin* and *neuraminidase* surface spikes, caused by the introduction of novel gene segments from the aquatic bird reservoir, that is responsible for pandemics of influenza.

genotype – The composition of gene segments in an influenza virus.

haemagglutinin (H) – The most prevalent protein on the surface of influenza virus that attaches to the cells of the respiratory tract and to the surface of red blood cells and makes them stick together (agglutinate).

haemagglutination inhibition (HI) – A test to detect antibodies to *haemagglutinin* that block the haemagglutinin on the virus from attaching to cells and thus provide protection from infection.

herd immunity – Resistance to the spread of a disease in the herd by immunity induced by exposure to that agent or vaccine to the disease agent.

interferons – A family of small *cytokine* proteins released by cells after infection with a disease agent that inhibit replication of the agent and provide the first line of defence.

lipid membrane – The surface proteins on the influenza virus particle, made up of fatty organic compounds acquired from the cell in which the virus multiplied.

live adapted influenza vaccine –Vaccine containing live influenza virus that has been 'cold adapted' to grow at 25°C but does not grow at normal body temperature (37°C). This vaccine is squirted up the nose of patients, where it multiplies at the lower temperature and induces protection.

macrophages – Large white blood cells found in body tissues and the bloodstream, which ingest and destroy invading organisms such as influenza viruses.

neuraminidase (N) – The second most prevalent protein on the surface of the influenza virus. This is an enzyme that releases the virus from the surface of infected cells and facilitates its spread.

neuraminidase inhibition test (NI) – A test to detect antibodies to the neuraminidase of the influenza virus that are induced after infection or vaccination and inhibit the spread of the virus.

nucleoprotein (NP) – A structural protein that surrounds the single-stranded *RNA* of a virus.

non-structural protein (NS1) – A protein that is encoded by a virus but is not included in the virus particle. The major role of NS1 is to shut down the antiviral response (e.g. *interferon* release) of the host to the virus.

pathogenic – Capable of causing disease.

peptides – Short chains of amino acids, held together by peptide bonds, that play a key role in regulating other molecules in cell function.

phagocytes – Cells in the body, such as *macrophages*, that protect against infection by ingesting invading agents and destroying them.

reassortment – The mixing of the genetic information of two viruses to produce a third. Influenza viruses have eight *RNA* segments. When any two different influenza viruses mix their genetic information, there are 256 different possible combinations.

reservoir – In disease research, this term refers to a natural storage place for disease agents. For influenza A viruses, reservoirs include populations of wild aquatic birds and bats.

RNA (ribonucleic acid) – The helical molecule that carries the genetic information of many viruses, including influenza viruses.

SARS (severe acute respiratory syndrome) – A contagious viral respiratory disease that can cause severe pneumonia and death. It is caused by a different group of viruses from influenza.

shedding – The release of influenza virus during sneezing or in saliva in mammals, or from faecal material from aquatic birds.

vaccine seed – The master strain of an influenza virus used for vaccine production. After WHO recommends an influenza virus be included in the seasonal vaccine, a seed stock is sent to vaccine manufacturers.

virus – A microscopic biological agent, consisting of a small amount of genetic material encased in protein, that reproduces in a living cell and may cause disease. An infected cell will rapidly produce thousands of copies of the original virus.

World Health Organization (WHO) – An agency of the United Nations, located in Geneva, Switzerland, concerned with international health. The Global Influenza Surveillance and Response System (GISRS) is the part of the WHO that monitors changes in influenza viruses throughout the world and makes recommendations on changes in influenza vaccines when warranted.

NOTES

1   E. Jordan, *Epidemic Influenza: A survey*, Chicago: American Medical Association, 1927.

2   A.W. Crosby Jr, *Epidemic and Peace, 1918*, Westport, Connecticut: Greenwood Press, 1976.

3   J.M. Barry, *The Great Influenza: The epic story of the deadliest plague in history*, New York: Penguin, 2004.

4   C.R. Byerly, *Fever of War: The influenza epidemic in the US Army during World War I*, New York: New York University Press, 2005.

5   G.M. Richardson, 'The onset of pneumonic influenza 1918 in relation to the wartime use of mustard gas', *NZMJ 47* (1948): 4–16.

6   A. Trilla, G. Trilla and C. Daer, 'The 1918 Spanish flu in Spain', *Clin Inf Dis 47* (2008): 668–73.

7   J.M. Barry, *The Great Influenza: The epic story of the deadliest plague in history*, New York: Penguin Books, 2004.

8   G.W. Rice, *Black November: The 1918 influenza pandemic in New Zealand* (2nd edn), Christchurch: Canterbury University Press, 2005.

9   G.W. Rice, *Black November*.

10 G.W. Rice, *Black November*.

11 T. Kessaram, J. Stanley and M.G. Baker, 'Estimating influenza-associated mortality in New Zealand from 1990 to 2008', *Influenza Other Respir Viruses 9(1)* (2015): 14–19.

12 N.A. Molinari, I.R. Ortega-Sanchez, M.L. Messonnier, W.W. Thompson, P.M. Wortley, E. Weintraub and C.B. Bridges, 'The annual impact of seasonal influenza in the US: Measuring disease burden and costs', *Vaccine 25(27)* (2007): 5086–96.

13 E. Centanni and E. Savonuzzi, 'La peste aviaria I & II', *Communicazione fatta all'accademia delle scienze mediche e naturali de Ferrara,* 1901.

14 W. Schäfer, 'Vergleichende sero-immunologische Untersuchungen über die Viren der Influenza und klassichen Geflügelpest' [Comparative sero-immunological investigations on the viruses of influenza and classic fowl plague], *Zeitschrift für Naturforschung 10b* (1955): 81–91.

15 J.S. Koen, 'A practical method for field diagnosis of swine disease', *Am J Vet Med 14* (1919): 468–70.

16 R.E. Shope, 'Swine influenza. I. Experimental transmission and pathology', *J Exp Med 54* (1931): 349–59; R.E. Shope, 'Swine influenza. III. Filtration experiments and etiology', *J Exp Med 54* (1931): 373–85.

17   D. Tyrrell, 'Discovery of influenza viruses', in K.G. Nicholson, R.G. Webster, A.J. Hay (eds), *Textbook of Influenza*, Oxford: Blackwell Science, 1998 (19–26).

18   W. Smith and C.V. Stuart-Harris, 'Influenza infection of man from the ferret', *Lancet 228* (1936): 121–23.

19   F.M. Burnet, 'Influenza virus on the developing egg. I. Changes associated with the development of an egg-passage strain of virus', *Br J Exp Path 17(4)* (1936): 282–93.

20   G.K. Hirst, 'The agglutination of red cells by allantoic fluid of chick embryos infected with influenza virus', *Science 94(2427)* (1941): 22–23.

21   G.K. Hirst, 'Adsorption of influenza hemagglutinins and virus by red blood cells', *J Exp Med 76(2)* (1942): 195–209.

22   D. Bucher and P. Palese, 'The biologically active proteins of influenza virus: Neuraminidase', in E.D. Kilbourne (ed.), *The Influenza Viruses and Influenza*, New York: Academic Press, 1975 (83–123).

23   T. Francis Jr., 'A new type of virus from epidemic influenza', *Science 92* (1940): 405–08.

24   A.M.-M. Payne, 'The influenza programme of WHO', *Bull Wld Hlth Org 8(5–6)* (1953): 755–92.

25   C.M. Chu, C.H. Andrewes and A.W. Gledhill, 'Influenza in 1948–1949', *Bull Wld Hlth Org 3* (1950): 187–214.

26   W.B. Becker, 'The morphology of tern virus', *Virology 20* (1963): 318–27.

27   W.G. Laver, 'From the Great Barrier Reef to a "cure" for the flu: Tall tales, but true', *Perspect Biol Med 47(4)* (2004): 590–96.

28   J.C. Downie and W.G. Laver, 'Isolation of a type A influenza virus from an Australian pelagic bird', *Virology 51(2)* (1973): 259–69.

29   R.G. Webster, M. Yakhno, V.S. Hinshaw, W.J. Bean and K.G. Murti, 'Intestinal influenza: Replication and characterization of influenza viruses in ducks', *Virology 84(2)* (1978): 268–78.

30   B.C. Easterday, D.O. Trainer, B. Tůmová and H.G. Pereira, 'Evidence of infection with influenza viruses in migratory waterfowl', *Nature 219(5153)* (1968): 523–24.

31   R.D. Slemons, D.C. Johnson, J.S. Osborn and F. Hayes, 'Type-A influenza viruses isolated from wild free-flying ducks in California', *Avian Dis 18(1)* (1974): 119–24.

32   R.G. Webster, M. Morita, C. Pridgen and B. Tůmová, 'Ortho- and paramyxoviruses from migrating feral ducks: Characterization of a new group of influenza A viruses', *J Gen Virol 32(2)* (1976): 217–25.

33   R.G. Webster, M. Yakhno, V.S. Hinshaw, W.J. Bean and K.G. Murti, 'Intestinal influenza: Replication and characterization of influenza viruses in ducks', *Virology 84(2)* (1978): 268–78.

34   V.S. Hinshaw, R.G. Webster and B. Turner, 'Novel influenza A viruses isolated from Canadian feral ducks: Including strains antigenically related to swine influenza (Hsw1N1) viruses', *J Gen Virol 41(1)* (1978): 115–27.

35 B. Harrington, *The Flight of the Red Knot*, New York/London: W.W. Norton and Co, 1996; D. Cramer, *The Narrow Edge: A tiny bird, an ancient crab and an epic journey*, New Haven, Connecticut: Yale University Press, 2015.

36 P. Hoose, *Moonbird: A year on the wing with the great survivor B95*, New York: Farrar, Straus and Giroux, 2012.

37 C.N. Shuster, H.J. Brockmann and R. Barlow (eds), *The American Horseshoe Crab*, Cambridge, Massachusetts/London: Harvard University Press, 2003.

38 I.L. Graves, 'Influenza viruses in birds of the Atlantic flyway', *Avian Diseases 36* (1992): 1–10.

39 Y. Kawaoka, T.M. Chambers, W.L. Sladen and R.G. Webster, 'Is the gene pool of influenza viruses in shorebirds and gulls different from that in wild ducks?', *Virology 163(1)* (1988): 247–50.

40 S. Krauss, D.E. Stallknecht, N.J. Negovetich, L.J. Niles, R.J. Webby and R.G. Webster, 'Coincident ruddy turnstone migration and horseshoe crab spawning creates an ecological "hot spot" for influenza viruses', *Proc Biol Sci 277(1699)* (2010): 3373–79.

41 Larry Niles, I.J. Niles and Associates, Rutgers University, personal communication.

42 L. Niles, J. Burger and A. Dey, *Life Along the Delaware Bay, Cape May: Gateway to a million shorebirds*, New Brunswick: Rivergate Books (Rutgers University Press), 2012.

43 B. Tůmová and B.C. Easterday, 'Relationship of envelope antigens of animal influenza viruses to human A2 influenza strains isolated in the years 1957–68', *Bull Wld Hlth Org 41(3)* (1969): 429–35.

44 H.G. Pereira, B. Tůmová and R.G. Webster, 'Antigenic relationship between influenza A viruses of human and avian origins', *Nature 215(5104)* (1967): 982–83.

45 R.G. Webster and H.G. Pereira, 'A common surface antigen in influenza viruses from human and avian sources', *J Gen Virol 3(2)* (1968): 201–08.

46 F.M. Burnet and P.E. Lind, 'Studies on recombination with influenza viruses in the chick embryo. III. Reciprocal genetic interaction between two influenza virus strains', *Aust J Exp Biol Med Sci 30(6)* (1952): 469–77.

47 Pereira, Tůmová and Webster, 'Antigenic relationship between influenza A viruses of human and avian origins'.

48 R.G. Webster, C.H. Campbell and A. Granoff, 'The "in vivo" production of "new" influenza A viruses. I. Genetic recombination between avian and mammalian influenza viruses', *Virology 44(2)* (1971): 317–28.

49 L.J. Zakstelskaja, N.A. Evstigneeva, V.A. Isachenko, S.P. Shenderovitch and V.A. Efimova, 'Influenza in the USSR: New antigenic variant A2-Hong Kong-1-68 and its possible precursors', *Am J Epidemiol 90(5)* (1969): 400–05.

50 W.G. Laver and R.G. Webster, 'Studies on the origin of pandemic influenza. III. Evidence implicating duck and equine influenza viruses as possible progenitors of the Hong Kong strain of human influenza', *Virology 51(2)* (1973): 383–91.

51   C.M. Chu, C. Shao, C.C. Hou, 'Studies of strains of influenza viruses isolated during the epidemic in 1957 in Changchun', *Vopr Virusol 2(5)* (1957): 278–81.

52   W. Chang, 'National influenza experience in Hong Kong, 1968', *Bull Wld Hlth Org 41(3)* (1969): 349–51.

53   S. Lui, 'An ethnographic comparison of wet markets and supermarkets in Hong Kong, 2008', *The Hong Kong Anthr 2* (2008): 1–52.

54   K.F. Shortridge, W.K. Butterfield, R.G. Webster and C.H. Campbell, 'Isolation and characterization of influenza A viruses from avian species in Hong Kong', *Bull Wld Hlth Org 55* (1977): 15–20.

55   K.F. Shortridge, R.G. Webster, W.K. Butterfield and C.H. Campbell, 'Persistence of Hong Kong influenza virus variants in pigs', *Science 196* (1977): 1454–55.

56   K.F. Shortridge, W.K. Butterfield, R.G. Webster and C.H. Campbell, 'Diversity of influenza A virus subtypes isolated from domestic poultry in Hong Kong', *Bull Wld Hlth Org 57(3)* (1979): 465–69.

57   D.K. L'vov, B. Easterday, R. Webster, A.A. Sazonov and N.N. Zhilina, ['Virological and serological examination of wild birds during the spring migrations in the region of the Manych Reservoir, Rostov Province'], *Vopr Virusol 4* (1977): 409–14. [In Russian.]

58   F.J. Austin and R.G. Webster, 'Evidence of ortho- and paramyxoviruses in fauna from Antarctica', *J Wildl Dis 29(4)* (1993): 568–71.

59   A.C. Hurt, Y.C. Su, M. Aban, H. Peck, H. Lau, C. Baas, Y.M. Deng, N. Spirason, P. Ellström, J. Hernandez, B. Olsen, I.G. Barr, D. Vijaykrishna and D. Gonzalez-Acuna, 'Evidence for the introduction, reassortment, and persistence of diverse influenza A viruses in Antarctica', *J Virol 90(21)* (2016): 9674–82.

60   N. Zhou, S. He, T. Zhang, W. Zou, L. Shu, G.B. Sharp and R.G. Webster, 'Influenza infection in humans and pigs in southeastern China', *Arch Virol 141(3–4)* (1996): 649–61.

61   L.L. Shu, N.N. Zhou, G.B. Sharp, S.Q. He, T.J. Zhang, W.W. Zou and R.G. Webster, 'An epidemiological study of influenza viruses among Chinese farm families with household ducks and pigs', *Epidemiol Infect 117(1)* (1996): 179–88.

62   J.C. de Jong, E.C. Claas, A.D. Osterhaus, R.G. Webster and W.L. Lim, 'A pandemic warning?', *Nature 389(6651)* (1997): 554.

63   K.F. Shortridge, N.N. Zhou, Y. Guan, P. Gao, T. Ito, Y. Kawaoka, S. Kodihalli, S. Krauss, D. Markwell, K.G. Murti, M. Norwood, D. Senne, L. Sims, A. Takada and R.G. Webster, 'Characterization of avian H5N1 influenza viruses from poultry in Hong Kong', *Virology 252(2)* (1998): 331–42.

64   L.D. Sims, T.M. Ellis, K.K. Liu, K. Dyrting, H. Wong, M. Peiris, Y. Guan and K.F. Shortridge, 'Avian influenza in Hong Kong 1997–2002', *Avian Dis 47(3 Suppl)* (2003): 832–38.

65   Y. Guan, K.F. Shortridge, S. Krauss and R.G. Webster, 'Molecular characterization of H9N2 influenza viruses: Were they the donors of the "internal" genes of H5N1 viruses in Hong Kong?', *Proc Natl Acad Sci USA 96(16)* (1999): 9363–67.

66   H. Chen, G. Deng, Z. Li, G. Tian, Y. Li, P. Jiao, L. Zhang, Z. Liu, R.G. Webster and K. Yu, 'The evolution of H5N1 influenza viruses in ducks in southern China', *Proc Natl Acad Sci USA 101(28)* (2004): 10452–57.

67   K.S. Li, Y. Guan, J. Wang, G.J. Smith, K.M. Xu, L. Duan, A.P. Rahardjo, P. Puthavathana, C. Buranathai, T.D. Nguyen, A.T. Estoepangestie, A. Chaisingh, P. Auewarakul, H.T. Long, N.T. Hanh, R.J. Webby, L.L. Poon, H. Chen, K.F. Shortridge, K.Y. Yuen, R.G. Webster and J.S. Peiris, 'Genesis of a highly pathogenic and potentially pandemic H5N1 influenza virus in eastern Asia', *Nature 430(6996)* (2004): 209–13.

68   X. Xu, K. Subbarao, N.J. Cox and Y. Guo, 'Genetic characterization of the pathogenic influenza A/Goose/Guangdong/1/96 (H5N1) virus: Similarity of its hemagglutinin gene to those of H5N1 viruses from the 1997 outbreaks in Hong Kong', *Virology 261(1)* (1999): 15–19.

69   Y. Guan, L.L. Poon, C.Y. Cheung, T.M. Ellis, W. Lim, A.S. Lipatov, K.H. Chan, K.M. Sturm-Ramirez, C.L. Cheung, Y.H. Leung, K.Y. Yuen, R.G. Webster and J.S. Peiris, 'H5N1 influenza: A protean pandemic threat', *Proc Natl Acad Sci USA 101(21)* (2004): 8156–61.

70   A.K. Boggild, L. Yuan, D.E. Low and A.J. McGeer, 'The impact of influenza on the Canadian First Nations', *Can J Public Health 102(5)* (2011): 345–48.

71   S.M. Flint, J.S. Davis, J.Y. Su, E.P. Oliver-Landry, B.A. Rogers, A. Goldstein, J.H. Thomas, U. Parameswaran, C. Bigham, K. Freeman, P. Goldrick and S.Y.C. Tong, 'Disproportionate impact of pandemic (H1N1) 2009 influenza on Indigenous people in the Top End of Australia's Northern Territory', *Med J Aust 192(10)* (2010): 617–22.

72   H.V. Fineberg, 'Pandemic preparedness and response: Lessons from the H1N1 influenza of 2009', *N Engl J Med 370(14)* (2014): 1335–42.

73   A. Vincent, L. Awada, I. Brown, H. Chen, F. Claes, G. Dauphin, R. Donis, M. Culhane, K. Hamilton, N. Lewis, E. Mumford, T. Nguyen, S. Parchariyanon, J. Pasick, G. Pavade, A. Pereda, M. Peiris, T. Saito, S. Swenson, K. Van Reeth, R. Webby, F. Wong and J. Ciacci-Zanella, 'Review of influenza A virus in swine worldwide: A call for increased surveillance and research', *Zoonoses and Public Health 61* (2014): 4–17.

74   G.J. Smith, D. Vijaykrishna, J. Bahl, S.J. Lycett, M. Worobey, O.G. Pybus, S.K. Ma, C.L. Cheung, J. Raghwani, S. Bhatt, J.S. Peiris, Y. Guan and A. Rambaut, 'Origins and evolutionary genomics of the 2009 swine-origin H1N1 influenza A epidemic', *Nature 459(7250)* (2009): 1122–25.

75   R. Gao, B. Cao, Y. Hu, Z. Feng, D. Wang, W. Hu, J. Chen, Z. Jie, H. Qiu, K. Xu, X. Xu, H. Lu, W. Zhu, Z. Gao, N. Xiang, Y. Shen, Z. He, Y. Gu, Z. Zhang, Y. Yang, X. Zhao, L. Zhou, X. Li, S. Zou, Y. Zhang, X. Li, L. Yang, J. Guo, J. Dong, Q. Li, L. Dong, Y. Zhu, T. Bai, S. Wang, P. Hao, W. Yang, Y. Zhang, J. Han, H. Yu, D. Li, G.F. Gao, G. Wu, Y. Wang, Z. Yuan and Y. Shu, 'Human infection with a novel avian-origin influenza A (H7N9) virus', *N Engl J Med 368(20)* (2013): 1888–97.

76   J.S. Peiris, 'Severe Acute Respiratory Syndrome (SARS)', *J Clin Virol 28(3)* (2003): 245–47.

77 Y. Guan, B.J. Zheng, Y.Q. He, X.L. Liu, Z.X. Zhuang, C.L. Cheung, S.W. Luo, P.H. Li, L.J. Zhang, Y.J. Guan, K.M. Butt, K.L. Wong, K.W. Chan, W. Lim, K.F. Shortridge, K.Y. Yuen, J.S. Peiris and L.L. Poon, 'Isolation and characterization of viruses related to the SARS coronavirus from animals in southern China', *Science 302(5643)* (2003): 276–78.

78 J. Pu, S. Wang, Y. Yin, G. Zhang, R.A. Carter, J. Wang, G. Xu, H. Sun, M. Wang, C. Wen, Y. Wei, D. Wang, B. Zhu, G. Lemmon, Y. Jiao, S. Duan, Q. Wang, Q. Du, M. Sun, J. Bao, Y. Sun, J. Zhao, H. Zhang, G. Wu, J. Liu and R.G. Webster, 'Evolution of the H9N2 influenza genotype that facilitated the genesis of the novel H7N9 virus', *Proc Natl Acad Sci USA 112(2)* (2015): 548–53.

79 Pu et al., 'Evolution of the H9N2 influenza genotype'.

80 J.C. Jones, S. Sonnberg, R.J. Webby and R.G. Webster, 'Influenza A (H7N9) virus transmission between finches and poultry', *Emerg Infect Dis 21(4)* (2015): 619–28.

81 S. Krauss, D.E. Stallknecht, R.D. Slemons, A.S. Bowman, R.L. Poulson, J.M. Nolting, J.P. Knowles and R.G. Webster, 'The enigma of the apparent disappearance of Eurasian highly pathogenic H5 clade 2.3.4.4 influenza A viruses in North American waterfowl', *Proc Natl Acad Sci USA 113(32)* (2016): 9033–38.

82 J.K. Taubenberger, A.H. Reid, A.E. Krafft, K.E. Bijwaard and T.G. Fanning, 'Initial genetic characterization of the 1918 "Spanish" influenza virus', *Science 275(5307)* (1997): 1793–96.

83 K. Duncan, *Hunting the 1918 Flu: One scientist's search for a killer virus*, Toronto: University of Toronto Press, 2003.

84 P. Davies, *Catching Cold: 1918's forgotten tragedy and the scientific hunt for the virus that caused it*, London: Michael Joseph, 1999.

85 P. Davies, *Catching Cold*.

86 G. Kolata, *Flu: The story of the great influenza pandemic of 1918 and the search for the virus that caused it*, New York: Farrar, Straus and Giroux, 1999.

87 G. Kolata, *Flu*.

88 J.K. Taubenberger, A.H. Reid, R.M. Lourens, R. Wang, G. Jin and T.G. Fanning, 'Characterization of the 1918 influenza virus polymerase genes', *Nature 437(7060)* (2005): 889–93.

89 Taubenberger, et al., 'Characterization of the 1918 influenza virus polymerase genes'.

90 T.M. Tumpey, C.F. Basler, P.V. Aguilar, H. Zeng, A. Solórzano, D.E. Swayne, N.J. Cox, J.M. Katz, J.K. Taubenberger, P. Palese and A. García-Sastre, 'Characterization of the reconstructed 1918 Spanish influenza pandemic virus', *Science 310(5745)* (2005): 77–80; C.F. Basler and P.V. Aguilar, 'Progress in identifying virulence determinants of the 1918 H1N1 and the Southeast Asian H5N1 influenza A viruses', *Antiviral Res 79(3)* (2008): 166–78.

91 D. Kobasa, S.M. Jones, K. Shinya, J.C. Kash, J. Copps, H. Ebihara, Y. Hatta, J.H. Kim, P. Halfmann, M. Hatta, F. Feldmann, J.B. Alimonti, L. Fernando, Y. Li, M.G. Katze, H. Feldmann and Y. Kawaoka, 'Aberrant innate immune response

in lethal infection of macaques with the 1918 influenza virus', *Nature 445(7125)* (2007): 319–23.

92 J.K. Taubenberger, A.H. Reid and T.G. Fanning, 'Capturing a killer flu virus', *Scientific American 292* (2005): 62–71.

93 C. Pappas, P.V. Aguilar, C.F. Basler, A. Solórzano, H. Zeng, L.A. Perrone, P. Palese, A. García-Sastre, J.M. Katz and T.M. Tumpey, 'Single gene reassortants identify a critical role for PB1, HA, and NA in the high virulence of the 1918 pandemic influenza virus', *Proc Natl Acad Sci USA 105(8)* (2008): 3064–69.

94 G.D. Shanks and J.F. Brundage, 'Pathogenic responses among young adults during the 1918 influenza pandemic', *Emerging Infectious Diseases 18* (2012): 201–07.

95 R.T. Ravenholt and W.H. Foege, '1918 influenza, encephalitis lethargica, parkinsonism', *Lancet 2(8303)* (1982): 860–64.

96 D. Kobasa, S.M. Jones, K. Shinya, J.C. Kash, J. Copps, H. Ebihara, Y. Hatta, J.H. Kim, P. Halfmann, M. Hatta, F. Feldmann, J.B. Alimonti, L. Fernando, Y. Li, M.G. Katze, H. Feldmann and Y. Kawaoka, 'Aberrant innate immune response in lethal infection of macaques with the 1918 influenza virus', *Nature 445(7125)* (2007): 319–23.

97 H. Jang, D. Boltz, K. Sturm-Ramirez, K.R. Shepherd, Y. Jiao, R. Webster and R.J. Smeyne, 'Highly pathogenic H5N1 influenza virus can enter the central nervous system and induce neuroinflammation and neurodegeneration', *Proc Natl Acad Sci USA 106(33)* (2009): 14063–68.

98 Taubenberger et al., 'Characterization of the 1918 influenza virus polymerase genes'.

99 Herfst et al., 'Airborne transmission of influenza A/H5N1 virus between ferrets'.

100 M. Imai, T. Watanabe, M. Hatta, S.C. Das, M. Ozawa, K. Shinya, G. Zhong, A. Hanson, H. Katsura, S. Watanabe, C. Li, E. Kawakami, S. Yamada, M. Kiso, Y. Suzuki, E.A. Maher, G. Neumann and Y. Kawaoka, 'Experimental adaptation of an influenza H5 HA confers respiratory droplet transmission to a reassortant H5 HA/H1N1 virus in ferrets', *Nature 486(7403)* (2012): 420–28.

BIBLIOGRAPHY

Austin, F.J. and R.G. Webster, 'Evidence of ortho- and paramyxoviruses in fauna from Antarctica', *J Wildl Dis 29(4)* (1993): 568–71.

Barry, J.M., *The Great Influenza: The epic story of the deadliest plague in history*, New York: Penguin, 2004.

Basler, C.F. and P.V. Aguilar, 'Progress in identifying virulence determinants of the 1918 H1N1 and the Southeast Asian H5N1 influenza A viruses', *Antiviral Res 79(3)* (2008): 166–78.

Becker, W.B., 'The morphology of tern virus', *Virology 20* (1963): 318–27.

Boggild, A.K., L. Yuan, D.E. Low and A.J. McGeer, 'The impact of influenza on the Canadian First Nations', *Can J Public Health 102(5)* (2011): 345–48.

Bucher, D. and P. Palese, 'The biologically active proteins of influenza virus: Neuraminidase', in E.D. Kilbourne (ed.), *The Influenza Viruses and Influenza*, New York: Academic Press, 1975 (83–123).

Burnet, F.M., 'Influenza virus on the developing egg. I. Changes associated with the development of an egg-passage strain of virus', *Br J Exp Path 17(4)* (1936): 282–93.

Burnet, F.M. and P.E. Lind, 'Studies on recombination with influenza viruses in the chick embryo. III. Reciprocal genetic interaction between two influenza virus strains', *Aust J Exp Biol Med Sci 30(6)* (1952): 469–77.

Byerly, C.R., *Fever of War: The influenza epidemic in the US Army during World War I*, New York: New York University Press, 2005.

Centanni, E. and E. Savonuzzi, 'La peste aviaria I & II', Communicazione fatta all'accademia delle scienze mediche e naturali de Ferrara, 1901.

Chang, W., 'National influenza experience in Hong Kong, 1968', *Bull Wld Hlth Org 41(3)* (1969): 349–51.

Chen, H., G. Deng, Z. Li, G. Tian, Y. Li, P. Jiao, L. Zhang, Z. Liu, R.G. Webster and K. Yu 'The evolution of H5N1 influenza viruses in ducks in southern China', *Proc Natl Acad Sci USA 101(28)* (2004): 10452–57.

Chu, C.M., C.H. Andrewes and A.W. Gledhill, 'Influenza in 1948–1949', *Bull Wld Hlth Org 3* (1950): 187–214.

Chu, C.M., C. Shao and C.C. Hou, 'Studies of strains of influenza viruses isolated during the epidemic in 1957 in Changchun', *Vopr Virusol 2(5)* (1957): 278–81.

Cramer, D., *The Narrow Edge: A tiny bird, an ancient crab and an epic journey*, New Haven, Connecticut: Yale University Press, 2015.

Crosby, A.W., *America's Forgotten Pandemic: The influenza of 1918*, Cambridge: Cambridge University Press, 1989, 295.

Crosby, A.W., *Epidemic and Peace, 1918*, Westport, Connecticut: Greenwood Press, 1976.

de Jong, J.C., E.C. Claas, A.D. Osterhaus, R.G. Webster and W.L. Lim, 'A pandemic warning?', *Nature 389(6651)* (1997): 554.

Downie, J.C. and W.G. Laver, 'Isolation of a type A influenza virus from an Australian pelagic bird', *Virology 51(2)* (1973): 259–69.

Duncan, K., *Hunting the 1918 flu: One scientist's search for a killer virus*, Toronto: University of Toronto Press, 2003.

Easterday, B.C., D.O. Trainer, B. Tůmová and H.G. Pereira, 'Evidence of infection with influenza viruses in migratory waterfowl', *Nature 219(5153)* (1968): 523–24.

Fineberg, H.V., 'Pandemic preparedness and response. Lessons from the H1N1 influenza of 2009', *N Engl J Med 370(14)* (2014): 1335–42.

Flint, S.M., J.S. Davis, J.Y. Su, E.P. Oliver-Landry, B.A. Rogers, A. Goldstein, J.H. Thomas, U. Parameswaran, C. Bigham, K. Freeman, P. Goldrick and S.Y.C. Tong, 'Disproportionate impact of pandemic (H1N1) 2009 influenza on indigenous people in the top end of Australia's Northern Territory', *Med J Aust 192(10)* (2010): 617–22.

Francis, T., Jr., 'A new type of virus from epidemic influenza', *Science 92* (1940): 405–08.

Gao, R., B. Cao, Y. Hu, Z. Feng, D. Wang, W. Hu, J. Chen, Z. Jie, H. Qiu, K. Xu, X. Xu, H. Lu, W. Zhu, Z. Gao, N. Xiang, Y. Shen, Z. He, Y. Gu, Z. Zhang, Y. Yang, X. Zhao, L. Zhou, X. Li, S. Zou, Y. Zhang, X. Li, L. Yang, J. Guo, J. Dong, Q. Li, L. Dong, Y. Zhu, T. Bai, S. Wang, P. Hao, W. Yang, Y. Zhang, J. Han, H. Yu, D. Li, G.F. Gao, G. Wu, Y. Wang, Z. Yuan and Y. Shu, 'Human infection with a novel avian-origin influenza A (H7N9) virus', *N Engl J Med 368(20)* (2013): 1888–97.

Graves, I.L., 'Influenza viruses in birds of the Atlantic flyway', *Avian Diseases 36* (1992): 1–10.

Guan, Y., L.L. Poon, C.Y. Cheung, T.M. Ellis, W. Lim, A.S. Lipatov, K.H. Chan, K.M. Sturm-Ramirez, C.L. Cheung, Y.H. Leung, K.Y. Yuen, R.G. Webster and J.S. Peiris, 'H5N1 influenza: A protean pandemic threat', *Proc Natl Acad Sci USA 101(21)* (2004): 8156–61.

Guan, Y., K.F. Shortridge, S. Krauss and R.G. Webster, 'Molecular characterization of H9N2 influenza viruses: Were they the donors of the "internal" genes of H5N1 viruses in Hong Kong?', *Proc Natl Acad Sci USA 96(16)* (1999): 9363–67.

Guan, Y., B.J. Zheng, Y.Q. He, X.L. Liu, Z.X. Zhuang, C.L. Cheung, S.W. Luo, P.H. Li, L.J. Zhang, Y.J. Guan, K.M. Butt, K.L. Wong, K.W. Chan, W. Lim, K.F. Shortridge, K.Y. Yuen, J.S. Peiris and L.L. Poon, 'Isolation and characterization of viruses related to the SARS coronavirus from animals in southern China', *Science 302(5643)* (2003): 276–78.

Harrington, B., *The Flight of the Red Knot*, New York/London: W.W. Norton and Co, 1996.

Herfst, S., E.J. Schrauwen, M. Linster, S. Chutinimitkul, E. de Wit, V.J. Munster, E.M. Sorrell, T.M. Bestebroer, D.F. Burke, D.J. Smith, G.F. Rimmelzwaan, A.D. Osterhaus and R.A. Fouchier, 'Airborne transmission of influenza A/H5N1 virus between ferrets', *Science 336(6088)* (2012): 1534–41.

Hinshaw, V.S., R.G. Webster and B. Turner, 'Novel influenza A viruses isolated from Canadian feral ducks: Including strains antigenically related to swine influenza (Hsw1N1) viruses', *J Gen Virol 41(1)* (1978): 115–27.

Hirst, G.K., 'Adsorption of influenza hemagglutinins and virus by red blood cells', *J Exp Med 76(2)* (1942): 195–209.

Hirst, G.K., 'The agglutination of red cells by allantoic fluid of chick embryos infected with influenza virus', *Science 94(2427)* (1941): 22–23.

Hoose, P., *Moonbird: A year on the wing with the great survivor B95*, New York: Farrar, Straus and Giroux, 2012.

Hurt, A.C., Y.C. Su, M. Aban, H. Peck, H. Lau, C. Baas, Y.M. Deng, N. Spirason, P. Ellström, J. Hernandez, B. Olsen, I.G. Barr, D. Vijaykrishna and D. Gonzalez-Acuna, 'Evidence for the introduction, reassortment, and persistence of diverse influenza A viruses in Antarctica', *J Virol 90(21)* (2016): 9674–82.

Imai, M., T. Watanabe, M. Hatta, S.C. Das, M. Ozawa, K. Shinya, G. Zhong, A. Hanson, H. Katsura, S. Watanabe, C. Li, E. Kawakami, S. Yamada, M. Kiso, Y. Suzuki, E.A. Maher, G. Neumann and Y. Kawaoka, 'Experimental adaptation of an influenza H5 HA confers respiratory droplet transmission to a reassortant H5 HA/H1N1 virus in ferrets', *Nature 486(7403)* (2012): 420–28.

Jang, H., D. Boltz, K. Sturm-Ramirez, K.R. Shepherd, Y. Jiao, R. Webster and R.J. Smeyne, 'Highly pathogenic H5N1 influenza virus can enter the central nervous system and induce neuroinflammation and neurodegeneration', *Proc Natl Acad Sci USA 106(33)* (2009): 14063–68.

Jones, J.C., S. Sonnberg, R.J. Webby and R.G. Webster, 'Influenza A (H7N9) virus transmission between finches and poultry', *Emerg Infect Dis 21(4)* (2015): 619–28.

Jordan, E., *Epidemic Influenza: A survey*, Chicago: American Medical Association, 1927.

Kawaoka, Y., T.M. Chambers, W.L. Sladen and R.G. Webster, 'Is the gene pool of influenza viruses in shorebirds and gulls different from that in wild ducks?', *Virology 163(1)* (1988): 247–50.

Kessaram, T., J. Stanley and M.G. Baker, 'Estimating influenza-associated mortality in New Zealand from 1990 to 2008', *Influenza Other Respir Viruses 9(1)* (2015): 14–19.

Kobasa, D., S.M. Jones, K. Shinya, J.C. Kash, J. Copps, H. Ebihara, Y. Hatta, J.H. Kim, P. Halfmann, M. Hatta, F. Feldmann, J.B. Alimonti, L. Fernando, Y. Li, M.G. Katze, H. Feldmann and Y. Kawaoka, 'Aberrant innate immune response in lethal infection of macaques with the 1918 influenza virus', *Nature 445(7125)* (2007): 319–23.

Koen, J.S., 'A practical method for field diagnosis of swine disease', *Am J Vet Med 14* (1919): 468–70.

Krauss, S., D.E. Stallknecht, N.J. Negovetich, L.J. Niles, R.J. Webby and R.G. Webster, 'Coincident ruddy turnstone migration and horseshoe crab spawning creates an ecological "hot spot" for influenza viruses', *Proc Biol Sci 277(1699)* (2010): 3373–79.

Krauss, S., D.E. Stallknecht, R.D. Slemons, A.S. Bowman, R.L. Poulson, J.M. Nolting, J.P. Knowles and R.G. Webster, 'The enigma of the apparent disappearance of Eurasian highly pathogenic H5 clade 2.3.4.4 influenza A viruses in North American waterfowl', *Proc Natl Acad Sci USA 113(32)* (2016): 9033–38.

L'vov, D.K., B. Easterday, R. Webster, A.A. Sazonov and N.N. Zhilina, ['Virological and serological examination of wild birds during the spring migrations in the region of the Manych Reservoir, Rostov Province'], *Vopr Virusol 4* (1977): 409–14. [In Russian.]

Laver, W.G., 'From the Great Barrier Reef to a "cure" for the flu: Tall tales, but true', *Perspect Biol Med 47(4)* (2004): 590–96.

Laver, W.G. and R.G. Webster, 'Studies on the origin of pandemic influenza. III. Evidence implicating duck and equine influenza viruses as possible progenitors of the Hong Kong strain of human influenza', *Virology 51(2)* (1973): 383–91.

Li, K.S., Y. Guan, J. Wang, G.J. Smith, K.M. Xu, L. Duan, A.P. Rahardjo, P. Puthavathana, C. Buranathai, T.D. Nguyen, A.T. Estoepangestie, A. Chaisingh, P. Auewarakul, H.T. Long, N.T. Hanh, R.J. Webby, L.L. Poon, H. Chen, K.F. Shortridge, K.Y. Yuen, R.G. Webster and J.S. Peiris, 'Genesis of a highly pathogenic and potentially pandemic H5N1 influenza virus in eastern Asia', *Nature 430(6996)* (2004): 209–13.

Lui, S., 'An ethnographic comparison of wet markets and supermarkets in Hong Kong, 2008', *The Hong Kong Anthr 2* (2008): 1–52.

Molinari, N.A., I.R. Ortega-Sanchez, M.L. Messonnier, W.W. Thompson, P.M. Wortley, E. Weintraub and C.B. Bridges, 'The annual impact of seasonal influenza in the US: Measuring disease burden and costs', *Vaccine 25(27)* (2007): 5086–96.

Niles, L., J. Burger and A. Dey, *Life Along the Delaware Bay, Cape May: Gateway to a million shorebirds*, New Brunswick: Rivergate Books (Rutgers University Press), 2012.

Pappas, C., P.V. Aguilar, C.F. Basler, A. Solórzano, H. Zeng, L.A. Perrone, P. Palese, A. García-Sastre, J.M. Katz and T.M. Tumpey, 'Single gene reassortants identify a critical role for PB1, HA, and NA in the high virulence of the 1918 pandemic influenza virus', *Proc Natl Acad Sci USA 105(8)* (2008): 3064–69.

Payne, A.M.-M., 'The influenza programme of WHO', *Bull Wld Hlth Org 8(5–6)* (1953): 755–92.

Peiris, J.S., 'Severe Acute Respiratory Syndrome (SARS)', *J Clin Virol 28(3)* (2003): 245–47.

Pereira, H.G., B. Tŭmová and R.G. Webster, 'Antigenic relationship between influenza A viruses of human and avian origins', *Nature 215(5104)* (1967): 982–83.

Pu, J., S. Wang, Y. Yin, G. Zhang, R.A. Carter, J. Wang, G. Xu, H. Sun, M. Wang, C. Wen, Y. Wei, D. Wang, B. Zhu, G. Lemmon, Y. Jiao, S. Duan, Q. Wang, Q. Du, M. Sun, J. Bao, Y. Sun, J. Zhao, H. Zhang, G. Wu, J. Liu and R.G. Webster, 'Evolution of the H9N2 influenza genotype that facilitated the genesis of the novel H7N9 virus', *Proc Natl Acad Sci USA 112(2)* (2015): 548–53.

Ravenholt R.T. and W.H. Foege, '1918 influenza, encephalitis lethargica, parkinsonism', *Lancet 2(8303)* (1982): 860–64.

Rice, G.W., *Black November: The 1918 influenza pandemic in New Zealand*, New Zealand: Allen & Unwin, 1988.

Rice, G.W., *Black November: The 1918 influenza pandemic in New Zealand* (2nd ed.), Christchurch: Canterbury University Press, 2005.

Richardson, G.M., 'The onset of pneumonic influenza 1918 in relation to the wartime use of mustard gas', *NZMJ 47* (1948): 4–16.

Schäfer, W., 'Vergleichende sero-immunologische Untersuchungen über die Viren der Influenza und klassichen Geflügelpest' [Comparative sero-immunological investigations on the viruses of influenza and classical fowl plague], *Zeitschrift für Naturforschung 10b* (1955): 81–91.

Shope, R.E., 'Swine influenza. I. Experimental transmission and pathology', *J Exp Med 54* (1931), 349–59

Shope, R.E., 'Swine influenza. III. Filtration experiments and etiology', *J Exp Med 54* (1931): 373–85.

Shortridge, K.F., W.K. Butterfield, R.G. Webster and C.H. Campbell, 'Diversity of influenza A virus subtypes isolated from domestic poultry in Hong Kong', *Bull Wld Hlth Org 57(3)* (1979): 465–69.

Shortridge, K.F., W.K. Butterfield, R.G. Webster and C.H. Campbell, 'Isolation and characterization of influenza A viruses from avian species in Hong Kong', *Bull Wld Hlth Org 55* (1977): 15–20.

Shortridge, K.F., R.G. Webster, W.K. Butterfield and C.H. Campbell, 'Persistence of Hong Kong influenza virus variants in pigs', *Science 196* (1977): 1454–55.

Shortridge, K.F., N.N. Zhou, Y. Guan, P. Gao, T. Ito, Y. Kawaoka, S. Kodihalli, S. Krauss, D. Markwell, K.G. Murti, M. Norwood, D. Senne, L. Sims, A. Takada and R.G. Webster, 'Characterization of avian H5N1 influenza viruses from poultry in Hong Kong', *Virology 252(2)* (1998): 331–42.

Shu, L.L., N.N. Zhou, G.B. Sharp, S.Q. He, T.J. Zhang, W.W. Zou and R.G. Webster, 'An epidemiological study of influenza viruses among Chinese farm families with household ducks and pigs', *Epidemiol Infect 117(1)* (1996): 179–88.

Shuster C.N., H. Jane Brockmann and R.B. Barlow (eds), *The American Horseshoe Crab*, Cambridge, Massachusetts/London: Harvard University Press, 2003.

Sims, L.D., T.M. Ellis, K.K. Liu, K. Dyrting, H. Wong, M. Peiris, Y. Guan and K.F. Shortridge, 'Avian influenza in Hong Kong 1997–2002', *Avian Dis 47(3 Suppl)* (2003): 832–38.

Slemons, R.D., D.C. Johnson, J.S. Osborn and F. Hayes, 'Type-A influenza viruses isolated from wild free-flying ducks in California', *Avian Dis 18(1)* (1974): 119–24.

Smith, G.J., D. Vijaykrishna, J. Bahl, S.J. Lycett, M. Worobey, O.G. Pybus, S.K. Ma, C.L. Cheung, J. Raghwani, S. Bhatt, J.S. Peiris, Y. Guan and A. Rambaut, 'Origins and evolutionary genomics of the 2009 swine-origin H1N1 influenza A epidemic', *Nature 459(7250)* (2009): 1122–25.

Smith, W. and C.V. Stuart-Harris, 'Influenza infection of man from the ferret', *Lancet* (1936): 121–23.

Taubenberger, J.K., A.H. Reid and T.G. Fanning, 'Capturing a killer flu virus', *Scientific American 292* (2005): 62–71.

Taubenberger, J.K., A.H. Reid, A.E. Krafft, K.E. Bijwaard and T.G. Fanning, 'Initial genetic characterization of the 1918 "Spanish" influenza virus', *Science 275(5307)* (1997): 1793–96.

Taubenberger, J.K., A.H. Reid, R.M. Lourens, R. Wang, G. Jin and T.G. Fanning, 'Characterization of the 1918 influenza virus polymerase genes', *Nature 437(7060)* (2005): 889–93.

Trilla, A., G. Trilla and C. Daer, 'The 1918 Spanish flu in Spain', *Clin Inf Dis 47* (2008): 668–73.

Tůmová, B. and B.C. Easterday, 'Relationship of envelope antigens of animal influenza viruses to human A2 influenza strains isolated in the years 1957–68', *Bull Wld Hlth Org 41(3)* (1969): 429–35.

Tumpey, T.M., C.F. Basler, P.V. Aguilar, H. Zeng, A. Solórzano, D.E. Swayne, N.J. Cox, J.M. Katz, J.K. Taubenberger, P. Palese and A. García-Sastre, 'Characterization of the reconstructed 1918 Spanish influenza pandemic virus', *Science 310(5745)* (2005): 77–80.

Tyrrell, D., 'Discovery of influenza viruses', in K.G. Nicholson, R.G. Webster and A.J. Hay (eds), *Textbook of Influenza*, Oxford: Blackwell Science, 1998 (19–26).

Vincent, A., L. Awada, I. Brown, H. Chen, F. Claes, G. Dauphin, R. Donis, M. Culhane, K. Hamilton, N. Lewis, E. Mumford, T. Nguyen, S. Parchariyanon, J. Pasick, G. Pavade, A. Pereda, M. Peiris, T. Saito, S. Swenson, K. Van Reeth, R. Webby, F. Wong and J. Ciacci-Zanella, 'Review of influenza A virus in swine worldwide: A call for increased surveillance and research',. *Zoonoses and Public Health 61* (2014): 4–17.

Webster, R.G., C.H. Campbell and A. Granoff, 'The "in vivo" production of "new" influenza A viruses. I. Genetic recombination between avian and mammalian influenza viruses', *Virology 44(2)* (1971): 317–28.

Webster R.G. and H.G. Pereira, 'A common surface antigen in influenza viruses from human and avian sources', *J Gen Virol 3(2)* (1968): 201–08.

Webster, R.G., M. Morita, C. Pridgen and B. Tůmová, 'Ortho- and paramyxoviruses from migrating feral ducks: Characterization of a new group of influenza A viruses', *J Gen Virol 32(2)* (1976): 217–25.

Webster, R.G., M. Yakhno, V.S. Hinshaw, W.J. Bean and K.G. Murti, 'Intestinal influenza: Replication and characterization of influenza viruses in ducks', *Virology 84(2)* (1978): 268–78.

Xu, X., K. Subbarao, N.J. Cox and Y. Guo, 'Genetic characterization of the pathogenic influenza A/Goose/Guangdong/1/96 (H5N1) virus: Similarity of its hemagglutinin gene to those of H5N1 viruses from the 1997 outbreaks in Hong Kong', *Virology 261(1)* (1999): 15–19.

Zakstelskaja, L.J., N.A. Evstigneeva, V.A. Isachenko, S.P. Shenderovitch and V.A. Efimova, 'Influenza in the USSR: New antigenic variant A2-Hong Kong-1-68 and its possible precursors', *Am J Epidemiol 90(5)* (1969): 400–05.

Zhou, N., S. He, T. Zhang, W. Zou, L. Shu, G.B. Sharp and R.G. Webster, 'Influenza infection in humans and pigs in southeastern China', *Arch Virol 141(3–4)* (1996): 649–61.

ACKNOWLEDGEMENTS

This book owes its existence to Marjorie, my wife, who not only raised three successful offspring while I chased viruses all over the world but also found the time to join in the search for influenza viruses on the beaches in Australia and United States, in the lakes in Canada and the poultry markets in Asia, and who is a fabulous wife and superb life companion. She supported every aspect of the work and taught me to always give something back.

The person who decided my life's work would be influenza research was the late Frank Fenner. As a graduate student I had moved to the Australian National University from New Zealand to work with him on the myxomatosis virus, which was being introduced to control the exploding rabbit population. I was chagrined when told that instead I would be conducting research on influenza with the late Stephen Fazekas de St Groth and Graeme Laver. As the book attests, however, the arrangement worked out rather well. A belated thank you to both Stephen and Graeme for marvellous mentoring.

Because many parts of the book were written from memory more than 50 years after the events occurred, it is inevitable that it includes some wishful thinking, as well as possible errors and omissions. I thank the many people who made the journey exciting but are not mentioned individually in these pages. Penny and Merran Laver, Jean Downie and Adrian Gibbs were of great help in digging through the records of trips to the Great Barrier Reef in Australia.

The privilege of spending six winter seasons at the University of Hong Kong with Ken Shortridge, Yi Guan and Malik Peiris in the Department of Microbiology from 1997 onwards also provided the opportunity for me to interact with Les Simms in the Department of Agriculture and Fisheries, Wilina Lim in the Health Department and many others. This experience gave me the opportunity for hands-on investigation of the human–animal interface during bird flu outbreaks. All these scientists contributed enormously to my understanding of the spread of influenza in live poultry markets and the difficulties faced by public health officials in control and prevention of the disease.

I am indebted to the many, many young people who provided ideas for lines of investigation and also did the grunt work in the field, at the bench and at the desk, writing the reports that made these studies possible: they have made me proud of their achievements at the influenza centres around the world. I also thank the Global Influenza Surveillance and Response System (GISRS) in the World Health Organization, which promotes the sharing of influenza viruses and knowledge and facilitated contacts and collaborations with brilliant people around the world. The studies were made possible by continuous support from the National Institutes of Health of the United States, which provided funding for over 50 years. The staff of the Canadian Wildlife Service, the Conserve Wildlife Foundation of New Jersey and the Endangered and Nongame Species Program of the New Jersey Division of Fish and Wildlife provided superior expertise and assistance for over four decades, making the wild bird studies possible.

St Jude Children's Research Hospital (SJCRH) and American Lebanese Syrian Associated Charities (ALSAC, the fundraising arm of SJCRH) provided support and the laboratory infrastructure and facilities. St Jude promotes interaction between scientists and physicians, emphasising the importance of control of infectious diseases during the treatment of childhood cancer. James Knowles and Elizabeth Stevens deserve special mention. James not only typed every draft and revision of this book but also corrected many details, while

Elizabeth Stevens provided the majority of the excellent diagrams.

The publishing team at Otago University Press were fantastic. Publisher Rachel Scott, with help from freelance editors Erika Büky and Sue Hallas, converted dry scientific details into readable text, and Rachel provided superb editing and encouragement throughout. Thanks to Fiona Moffat for the book's design, and Diane Lowther for the very thorough index.

For additional assistance in bringing the book to publication I am indebted to many scientific colleagues, including Lance Jennings, Maria Zambon, Geoffrey Rice, Michael Baker, Masato Tashiro, Bernard Easterday and the two anonymous peer reviewers who read and made valuable suggestions and corrections to the manuscript. Richard Webby, Paul Thomas and Keiji Fukuda reviewed multiple chapters during the early stages of writing and made invaluable comments, particularly on the immunology, 2009 H1N1 pandemic and international relationships.

The person who actually persuaded me to put pen to paper was Sharon Webster, my daughter-in-law; she pointed out in 2016, when I was vacillating about whether to attempt this book, that 2018 would mark the centennial of the 1918 Spanish influenza pandemic, and that surely I could not let that occasion pass without recounting the search for the origin of the monster virus in wild aquatic birds. Being an artist as well as a scientist, Sharon also designed the striking cover for the book.

INDEX

Page numbers in **bold** refer to illustrations.